REVOLUTIONARY HEALTH

James Loomis

REVOLUTIONARY HEALTH
_IS....._

- ❖ A plan for remission from cancer, heart disease and diabetes.

- ❖ A new way of thinking, speaking, eating and drinking.

- ❖ Your path to freedom from the bondage of obesity.

- ❖ A 9-step plan to put disease into remission.

- ❖ A book of hope, encouragement and action on how to live drug free and healthy.

- ❖ Your new life through easy to follow changes in perception and everyday activities.

- ❖ Freedom from pain, illness and diets.

- ❖ A plan of 11 points to prevent heart disease.

- ❖ Easy to follow with rewards of renewed strength, vitality and endurance.

- ❖ THE life you have always wanted.

- ❖ The way of the future.

This book is for informational purposes that are intended to be general advice on health care; it is not intended to be a substitute for medical advice of a licensed physician. The author is not a medical professional and nothing in this publication constitutes medical advice.

Any exercise program, including any exercise routines outlined in this publication, may result in injury. Any fitness program contains inherent risks of physical injury or death; always consult your physician prior to beginning any new exercise program to reduce the risk of injury. The information in this book is meant to supplement, not replace, proper training. The author advises readers to take full responsibility for their safety and know their limits.

This book is not intended as a substitute for doctor's advice, professional diagnosis, opinion, and treatment or services to you or to any other individual; it is presented AS IS. Always consult your doctor for your individual needs relating to your health, and regarding any symptoms that may require diagnosis or medical attention.

The author and publisher are not liable or responsible for any advice, course of treatment, diagnosis or any other information you obtain.

IF YOU BELIEVE YOU HAVE A MEDICAL EMERGENCY, YOU SHOULD IMMEDIATELY CALL 911 OR YOUR PHYSICIAN.

Revolutionary Health

ISBN 9781731556448

Copyright 2018 by James and Janie Loomis

Atlanta, Texas 75551

Printed in the United States of America

Cover artwork and layout by Janie Loomis

Other Books by James and Janie Loomis

- The 10-Day Total Body Revolution

- 30 Days to a Healthy Spirit, Soul and Body

- Passionate Lover of God

- The Spirit of the Forerunner: A Cry Goes Out

- The Spirit of the Forerunner: The Legacy of One Who Has Gone Before

- The Spirit of the Forerunner: Mantles of Our Predecessors

- Empower the Forerunner Within You
  Study Guide

➢ Empower the Forerunner Within You

    Workbook and Journal

➢ Empower the Forerunner Within You

    Teachers Edition

For a growing list of on-line workshops and interactive courses you can take to further your *Revolution* in spirit, soul and body visit our website listed below.

Additional copies of this book or other books of the authors may be obtained via their website or Amazon and Amazon Kindle. You may also attend one of their conferences or seminars to pick up copies of books or Forerunner Merchandise. To schedule a speaking engagement, or contact the author, visit the website or send us a direct email:

www.forerunnerspirit.com

forerunnerspirit@gmail.com

Table of Contents

Bonus Material

Dedication

This book is dedicated to my family

To my grandparents: although I did not know you
very well, nor had much time with you, through
you and your parents I am what I am.

To my parents: James and Genevieve thank you for
a wonderful childhood. Thank you for wanting,
loving and providing for me during my formative
years. Who I became is because of your inspiration,
guidance, instruction and patience with me. To be
called your son, I am truly honored.

To my wife Janie: you are my life. Being with
you for 40 years now has been incredible. All we
have experienced, the places we have visited and
lived, the hard work we have shared, the ups and
downs; life has not been easy but it has been
memorable. Through your consistent
encouragement, being a living example of a
Forerunner and co-worker in EVERY project I
have begun you have demonstrated incredible
stamina, direction, stability, and most of all love
beyond belief.

You have been, are and forever shall be the only
love of my life.

To my Heavenly Father:
Thank you for my life.

—

INTRODUCTION:

MY REVELATION TO REVOLUTION

I have not always held *Revolutionary* ideas. When I was young I was painfully shy and reclusive. There are times now I sometimes would prefer to be alone rather than addressing a crowd or counseling people one-on-one.

Slowly, over the years my self-confidence began to grow, probably because being married to an outgoing, gregarious, woman I started to view life differently. When asked as a young person, "what do you want to do when you grow up", I always responded, "I want to help people."

With my innate nature to help, I embarked in college in creative writing and reporting thinking that perhaps a field in Journalism would satisfy my need to research an event or cause and then report my findings to "help people."

In college I decided on a career in accounting thinking this profession could help individuals and companies in their finances. Over the years I have assisted countless individuals and firms in their economic well being; yet I still felt there was more.

When I became a Christian, I bought innumerable books on a wide variety of subjects, enrolled in classroom education classes and attended many seminars. Later I would assist in various capacities in the churches I attended and felt I was making a difference in "helping people."

And yet, still I have felt: there must be more I could do!

Throughout my life I have slowly self-restricted my eating and drinking habits as I have researched and learned the dangers of various types of foods.

Since the 1980's Janie and I have not eaten shellfish. In 2006 I began taking food preparation and food safety classes in relation to our restaurant and gourmet foods manufacturing business. It was during this time that I learned the extreme dangers of consuming shellfish; needless to say we still do not consume these products.

In the mid 1990's we stopped eating pork. We visited individual farms and corporations that raised hogs, witnessed first-hand the deplorable living conditions and parasite infestation. It was an easy decision to remove any of these products from our "menu" of approved foods.

Since opening our restaurant I have researched diseases, natural supplements, spices, the nutritional content of foods and so much more. I have reported my findings as a newspaper columnist, in seminars, conferences, in on-line discussion groups and individual counseling.

This is where I have now found my "more". I combine my ever-increasing knowledge and research in medicine and alternative practices with my faith and have been able to reach people who have been mistreated by traditional medicine and faith based groups. I demonstrate proven, practical and effective methods and procedures for healthy living and soul healing.

My life has slowly evolved to the point where I extremely, willingly restrict my food and drink intake and exhibit a lifestyle of health, wholeness and balance. This has proven exceptionally effective to those looking to alter their unhealthy lives.

I live a new life today; a *Revolutionary* lifestyle compared to most people I encounter. This new life can be yours today if you desire.

The rewards are astronomical in the plethora of new habits that heal our bodies and souls. I encourage you to join me in this journey to *Revolutionary Health*; it is really easier than you can imagine.

Never give up!
Never give in!
Never say die!

CHAPTER 1

NEVER GIVE UP

Now is the time, today is the day to change your life!

To be a *Revolutionary* you must act like a *Revolutionary*, talk like a *Revolutionary* and BELIEVE like a *Revolutionary*.

When you *Never Give Up* on yourself, on your family, on your profession, on your health and anything or anyone you prove to yourself first and foremost that you are not a quitter. You prove that you can go the distance. You prove that you can and will do what you set your mind, heart, spirit, soul and body to accomplish.

There are many great quotes, sayings and books you can read on this subject. Get yourself charged up that nothing will hold you back from undertaking and completing your specific goals. There are lots of great motivational speakers from whom you can glean much wisdom. When you find a quote that grabs you, I mean REALLY GRABS you, print it out and post it everywhere!

Think about it, no matter what you are doing, there is always a solution to your problem. You may not like the best solution, but it is there; you just need to discover what it is for your specific situation. Do not despair; get help if you need it. Read this book over and over and you will discover solutions.

You will be successful in your endeavours, it is inevitable, if you utilize wisdom, common sense, seek out those who may assist you and you Never Give Up!

Remember, you control your life circumstances. If you feel you are losing control or have no control over life events then you need to change the parameters of what you are doing. Alter conditions, environments and situations so you may regain control. Then take charge and get your life back.

Remember, your life has purpose and meaning. Through your experiences you become aware of your strengths and weaknesses and can awaken the "real you" that may be sleeping. You were born so you have a purpose for existence, the discovery of whom you are will propel you towards a meaningful life.

REDIRECT

When you believe you have done EVERYTHING you think you know to do and still nothing seems to work or problems exist, it is time to get real.

You need to re-evaluate: what you are doing, how you think, your self-picture, where you see your life going and your circle of friends. Get brutal with yourself, not demeaning but completely realistic.

Just because you may have had a bankruptcy in your past does not mean you are a loser. If you are divorced does not mean you are terrible with interpersonal relationships. Even though you have left one church for another does not mean you are a troublemaker.

BECAUSE you have a failure in your past and you are still moving forward is evidence that you have not given up on yourself or life circumstances. Sure, we all have problems and difficulties; the overcomer sees beyond their current circumstances to a future that is hopeful and filled with potential.

Now that you have "gotten real with yourself", let's make a number of declarations to insure your *Never Giving Up* status and put into the forefront of our brain some reminders on how to *Never Give Up*.

<u>VERBAL DECLARATIONS</u>

This may sound silly, odd, stupid, and nonsensical or any other term you want to say, but making a verbal declaration creates change on a multitude of levels.

When you hear your declaration, in your voice it goes into your ears and then to your mind and soul at a level you can grasp and hold onto better than just the reading the words on a page.

As these declarations go out into the atmosphere they carry a kind of power that aids them in coming to pass. Positive spoken words carry a power that aids them in coming into reality. Negative words carry similar power, so choose your words wisely.

Recite the following declarations out loud. Get excited with what you read. Put the declarations into practice. If you are not physically, financially or mentally able to put them into practice, start with what you can and work towards being able to believe and do the rest as soon as possible.

As you read these pronouncements, start thinking of your own personal declarations that you need to make. Write your affirmations or testimonials in this book so you have them to reference later.

Whatever it takes   ***I WILL NEVER GIVE UP***!

I have a purpose in life.

I am an inspiration to others.

I seek to be happy every day.

Because of ME the world is a better place.

I will succeed because I have everything I need.

The negativity of others will not hold me back.

I am almost there; I will not stop moving forward.

I have yet to try everything. There must be more.

Past failures do not determine my future.

I will not allow anyone or anything to divert me from the task I have appointed for myself.

I am beautifully and wonderfully created; I am a blessing to many people and many more who just do not know me yet.

<u>*I WILL NEVER GIVE UP!*</u>

----Now, right now, right here inscribe in this book declarations you make with yourself to yourself and to the world. ---

<u>**REMINDERS**</u>

We must change our thinking, our thought processes from that of defeatism to winning and overcoming. This is accomplished by unlearning what we have been taught in areas that are counterproductive to life and healing. I have had to do this repeatedly in many areas of my life over the years.

Then we must learn to think positively, not become jaded or cynical, but to speak good things to people from a mind that conjectures life differently than we have previously.

This is the *Revolutionary* way of life. We must deconstruct our past, learn from it, remember what we were taught, but move forward with a revised way of thinking, believing and acting. I acknowledge the truth of my circumstances, yet I profess that I will not remain in my current state of being.

As a *Revolutionary* <u>I modify</u> the circumstances of my life, I do not allow outside forces to alter my beliefs, practices and self-image. If I am, for example, overweight then as a *Revolutionary* I will be honest with myself, look within myself to determine why I am overweight, and then ***I*** make the determination what needs to be done to alter my life situation.

When you determine to do something, follow through with it. You must make YOU a priority in your life.

"Our greatest weakness lies in giving up. The most certain way to succeed is always to try just one more time." —THOMAS EDISON

<u>**CONCLUSION**</u>

Revolutionaries alter society by first becoming altered. Think about people who, by their words and deeds, have *revolutionized* the world. Begin with yourself, speak out your decrees and follow through with them. Put them on pieces of paper and tape them up all over your home. Put your decrees on your refrigerator, your bathroom mirror; put your decrees anywhere and everywhere throughout your house.

Believe in yourself. Do not give in to self-doubt, fear, or false beliefs that would attempt to hold you back.

Allow your mind, heart and soul to be changed to believe that you can change for good that you can change your world and YOU are the change agent.

Believe in yourself.

<u>***NEVER GIVE UP!***</u>

CHAPTER 2

NEVER GIVE IN

There are some things that are healthy for you to give in to, such as helping people, spreading love, encouraging those that are downcast, providing positive motivation and lending your strength and courage to those in need. There are many others, but these are a good start.

Do not give in to mentors that try to abuse and control you. Do not give in to sorrow or greed or lust or envy or passions that destroy your spirit, soul or body.

Never give in to sorrow or grief that may lead you to eat bad foods; which lead to obesity and a multitude of diseases. Never give in to feelings that cause depression and make you think you need to take psychotropic drugs.

Psychotropic and psychoactive drugs change brain functioning that result in alterations in perception, mood, consciousness, cognition or behaviour. If you give in to the "advise" or pressure of doctors or "well-meaning persons" who say you need to take these types of medications you will be changed.

It is *your choice* whether or not to take various drugs. There are alternative methods other than brain-altering substances that can deal with the wide variety of conditions for which medical practitioners prescribe these medications.

Always get a second or third medical opinion prior to settling on a course of medical treatment. Never give in to only one diagnosis and method of dealing with a physiological, spiritual or emotional problem.

Revolutionaries do not give in to outside pressures to conform to standard practices or procedures; they think for themselves and find better ways to overcome any obstacle presented to them.

ALTERED STATES OF BEING

You have already decided not to give up on yourself and to change your thinking process. Now you determine to never give in to outside forces, people, places or events that would misdirect you from what you have determined is best for your life.

Through your altered state of being, you determine to understand your health: physical, mental, emotional and spiritual, and as such your life takes on a whole new purpose, perspective and direction. This "altered state" is that of realization that you do not need drugs, some guru, the latest diet pill or crazy pseudo-science therapy to change your life, you only need determination and self-will.

You can change yourself and your world if you *Never Give In* to outside pressure to conform. You change by understanding yourself, why you act and react the way you do and then you change what needs to be changed.

Educate yourself, do not give in to group or peer pressures, see yourself as healthy emotionally, spiritually and physically and keep going strong no matter what is thrown at you.

You can alter your "state of being" through your will power to be different and the subsequent follow through to better yourself. It takes determination, being true to yourself and never giving in to voices that try to steer you off the path you should travel.

<u>WHY YOU SHOULD NEVER GIVE IN</u>

If you give in you may never realize everything that you were created to achieve. What is it that which would cause you to give in, to give up, to stop moving forward, to not care anymore? Analyse what makes you tick and would make you do something that you would regret later.

Do not give in to sorrow, to grief, to being motivated by guilt, to cravings for foods that kill your body, to relationships that harm your soul, those tear at your insides while all along you know you should not do something yet you do it anyway.

DO what is good and helpful, do what pushes you onward to be a better person and improves the lives of those around you. Sow peace, inspiration and dedication into YOUR life, as seeds into the soil, and reap a harvest that you can speak into the lives of those with whom you come into contact.

Be your own best friend. Take care of YOUR body first, and then seek to help others achieve ultimate health and welfare. If you are falling apart, how can you help others to reach their full potential?

These are a few of the opening reasons why you should never give in, but keep pressing forward with your life.

The following are a number of quick inspirational thoughts, or what I like to call proclamations. These are in the personal tense so you can keep motivated and encourage others. Speak these out loud as you read them.

--I am still alive, I am breathing so it is never too late to change and better myself. I am worth it. Anything is possible. The world needs me.

--I believe in myself. I believe in my dreams. I will follow though with what I feel is right for me to do.

--I have everything I need to succeed within me. I will examine myself, pull out what is needed and move forward with my life.

--I will allow no one, no event, or no thing to hold me back. I will succeed and accomplish my goals.

--I have no regret for the past. I acknowledge the past is the past and I cannot change it. I am learning from past mistakes and failures but I also learn from past victories and successes. I choose to succeed from now on and going forward in my life.

--I will no longer give up on myself nor give in to what held me back in the past.

--I do not need to prove myself to anyone. I am who I am; I strive to better myself but I recognize that I am who I am.

--I will succeed. I will overcome. I will be victorious.

--Regardless of current circumstances, though they may be difficult, I will press forward and not give in nor stop what I am doing.

--It is my destiny to be an inspiration to those around me, to make a difference in society and live in this moment of time.

--I am stronger than I think.

--What I do I do with excellence.

--I will never stop learning. I will continue to educate myself in the areas that are most meaningful to me.

--I deserve to be happy.

--I deserve to succeed.

--I may fail over and over and over again; I will pick myself up, wipe away my tears, get up, get going and never stop trying again and again and again!

--When someone says something cruel or mean or negative to me I will not return evil for evil. I will not allow their wickedness to become a part of me. I will not allow their words power over me or to destroy me.

--By my determination and focus on my goals I will succeed in what I do.

--I now stand at the threshold of the tipping point of my life. I am about to breakthrough into a new "realm" of life that permanently alters me to be a success, to be inspirational, to be all that I was created to become. I will not allow this moment to pass me by. I will step over that threshold and live MY new life.

<u>CONCLUSION</u>

Never give in to <u>anything</u> that would hold you back. Copy and paste the proclamations in this chapter anywhere and everywhere to keep you inspired to believe and do what you are destined to do.

Do not stop.

<u>NEVER GIVE IN!</u>

CHAPTER 3

NEVER SAY DIE

When you have a <u>Never Say Die</u> attitude it flows into every arena of your life. Your words, your actions and how you carry yourself. You are not arrogant or proud, but uplifting, joyful and positive. You are real you are not fake.

You are not discouraged over the long term. Life events may cause you to become disappointed, but you do not live in that emotion. Rather you pick yourself up, brush yourself off and ask yourself what am I learning from this incident? When you discover the intent of people's words and actions you can adjust your life accordingly; within kindness, love, patience and peace you reside so the long-term ill effects of others do not cause havoc to your life.

<u>**YOUR NEW YOU**</u>

As you are reading this book you are becoming a new person. You are becoming aware of feelings and emotions, thoughts and desires that were buried and are now coming to the surface. This is the real you striving to come forth.

The REAL you, the healthy you, the *Revolutionary* you is coming to the surface of your consciousness, permeating every aspect of your being. Allow this fresh wind, a new attitude, and a new perspective on life to be birthed within you. This "birthing" is the real you that is deep inside you that has always wanted and needed to be revealed.

According to the Merriam-Webster Dictionary:

<u>**never say die**</u>

 is an idiom—which means it is a group of words established by useage as having a meaning not deductible from those of the individual words.

That means: an idiom is a <u>phrase</u> that is greater than the indivdual words and carries a strong message (in this case) for the reader to draw inspiration, guidance, encouragement, strength and power.

Actual definition of *never say die*

—it is used to encourage someone to continue something or to remain hopeful.

With that background, let's take ourselves to the next level.

YOUR NEW *NEVER SAY DIE* ATTITUDE

You do not get discouraged, no matter what happens. No matter what "they" say or do to you. You are not a quitter. You are a fighter! You cannot be stopped!

When you are at a work-sponsored meal you stick to your *Revolutionary Health* protocol and choose to eat foods that are healthy or you do not eat at all. When you are out with your friends and everyone is drinking alcohol you remember your *Never Say Die* attitude and you do not drink.

You are the example setter: you are the one to whom everyone looks to see if you will be true to your beliefs or fail miserably. You are the leader that those at work, at school, in your church or social groups turn to when they want clear, direct answers without compromise or game playing.

You are an optimist. Good things are possible to happen not bad things inevitable to occur. You choose to reroute situations so you have choices, not get stuck in a position where you settle for second best.

You acknowledge your weaknesses, yet you strive to improve yourself and ask for advice. You search out positive outcomes to your health problems; you get multiple medical diagnoses before you settle on a course of action.

You believe in yourself. You keep practicing, you keep rehearsing, you study more, and you work out longer and harder than you have before. You are infectious.

Your life is a journey of which there have been many ups and downs, but you focus on what you have learned and you grow stronger and wiser. You do not beat yourself up over your mistakes and problems; you look forward to the next adventure.

No matter the odds that are stacked against you and regardless of the size of the task you are tenacious and overcome all obstacles. You press forward to win.

You know that if you give up on your dream, the dream will die. You press forward with a good attitude, a smile on your face, an encouraging word to all who see you and you maintain a pure, devoted heart. You will achieve your dream because you know within the very core of your being you will:

NEVER SAY DIE!

CONCLUSION

Being steadfast in your beliefs and convictions you will not be swayed or turned from the path you have chosen for your life. Being confident in yourself you do not allow people to guilt or cajole you into doing something you know is not healthy or right for you to do.

When others around you lose heart, get despondent or depressed and want to give up and quit you are the encourager that keeps them going. By your leadership qualities and the example you set, people are inspired and follow you.

Do not conform or bow to pressures to accept standards that are not what you hold dear to your heart. Reveal your uniqueness and character by adhereing to your plans and objectives while not pressuring anyone else to conform to your ways.

You allow people to make their own decisions, yet you live the life that **they** want to emulate. Stand your ground; do not be nervous or afraid for there is nothing to fear.

Be the *Revolutionary* to everyone you encounter by the way you talk, act, believe and carry yourself. Through your selfless mannerisms and actions you prove that you will:

NEVER GIVE UP!

NEVER GIVE IN!

NEVER SAY DIE!

CHAPTER 4

HEALING NOT MANAGING

Now is the time for you to be healed from any illness or condition, not just to "manage" your health as the health care profession advocates. If you TRULY want to be healed or cured of what ails you, you will do *Revolutionary* acts to make it happen.

I make no claims to heal or cure you of your condition by your following the admonitions and suggestions within this book; however I will say you may get closer to healing than what traditional medicine advocates.

Medicine is not magic nor is it 100% effective. There are doctors and hospitals that are "quacks" in their traditional medical practices as there are in alternative medicine. I applaud and recommend multiple diagnoses for medical conditions from a wide variety of professionals. This way you can make as qualified of decisions as possible.

DO YOUR RESEARCH

I have read countless books, Ebooks, and newspaper articles, analysed numerous research papers and medical studies, and downloaded file cabinets full of articles from a wide variety of sources on all types of medical procedures and alternative therapies. The Selected Bibliography at the end of this book will list a few of these sources for the suggestions I propose.

I encourage you to do your own research. Allow yourself the opportunity to try alternative medical programs. Always refer to a **_trusted_** medical adviser when starting any new program. Your body may react differently to procedures suggested in this book than may normally be the case due to your uniqueness and medical history.

Use common sense when approaching a lifestyle alteration. I hate the commercials that state their particular regimen of pills, shots, powders, drinks, or meals will **manage** your medical condition or bring your body into proper alignment and complete health. Be wary of and avoid "certified health specialists" who only want to sell you their line of pyramid scheme products.

Manufacturers and charlatans want you to take their pills and potions and pre-packaged, pre-measured meals for the rest of your life (how ever short it will be because of the side effects of this treatment). In reality your medical condition will not change because of their false advertisements, please remember the admonitions of the first three chapters of this book.

Manufacturers want repeat business. My wife and I wanted repeat customers when we manufactured and sold our line of gourmet foods. A customer likes one product, decides to try another and tells all their friends about the item. Drug manufacturers do not care if you "like" a drug or not, they want to control your life or **manage** your condition so you are addicted to their drugs and take them for the rest of your life.

Let me provide a caveat here, if you need a drug to live, I am not telling you to stop taking it or to go against the advice of your medical professional. What I am saying is if you do not want to take a certain drug or follow a particular regimen then do your own research and discover alternative therapies that may work for you.

First-remember the admonitions of chapters one through three of this book, second-think about, pray about, and do something different. If you want to lose weight, most of us have tried multiple plans, which is good, in this way you see how they do or do not work for you and your lifestyle. By investigating the creator of the diet, their tips and techniques you learn more about the creator(s) and if their plan may be good for you.

Most diets fail, because we cannot or will not follow through with the guidelines or they are actually harmful to our overall well-being. I believe we also need a paradigm shifting away from how we used to think and believe to actually achieve long-lasting success.

PARADIGM SHIFTING

My wife Janie was in medical trouble. She went a number of times to see our doctor and to the Emergency Room due to her medical condition and still did not have the answers to why she was in so much pain. Finally when our doctor said the pain was "just in her head" and she needed to take an anti-depressant drug, she knew it was time for a drastic change.

Eventually she was led to an Internal Medicine specialist who had some detailed blood tests done to find out that she had Hyperthyroidism. He said people have died going through what she had prior to seeing him.

The Internal Medicine doctor gave her three options: 1: Surgery to remove her thyroid gland 2: Radiation treatment to kill her thyroid gland or 3: Take pills. A lump had developed on her gland and it had to go one way or the other. If she chose either option 1 or 2 she would have to take pills for the rest of her life because then she would have hypothyroidism. To Janie, she had no options.

Janie started taking a tiny fraction of the pill the doctor recommended and then researched what herbs and spices would kill cancerous tumours. She started an intense regime of Pau d' arco, radically different eating habits (most foods gave her extreme intestinal distress) and the tiny portion of the medication.

In time her thyroid gland recovered! She still takes Pau d' arco, not as much as she used to take, but no longer needs the medication. She did not submit to surgery or radiation therapy and she recovered. The Pau d' arco killed the tumour that was growing on her thyroid gland!

Your story may be different than Janie's, however learn from her ordeal. She would not give in to a bad diagnosis. She would not give up researching how she could be healed naturally. She would not say-I am going to die from this medical problem-she said I will not die I will FIGHT with everything I have and I will overcome! She is a champion. She is victorious in her determination to do what she needed to do to overcome a life-threatening situation.

I remember how the actor Steve McQueen had fought with cancer using alternative therapies. He would not listen to traditional medical doctors but wanted to try radically different procedures. He knew the risks, but he was willing to try. I commend him for going beyond what was presented to him and trying something different to see if it would help.

I know of people who were diagnosed with a terminal illness and volunteered to participate in medical drug trials and testing. These drugs or surgical procedures could backfire and kill the person or perhaps help save more lives later. The people who underwent these trials were brave and to the end believed if others could be helped through what they would go through then it would be worth the pain and suffering.

Are you ready to make your paradigm shift, to become a *Revolutionary*? Are you ready and willing to move beyond trying to **manage** a physical or mental or emotional situation and actually become healed of WHATEVER is going on in your life? If so, then let's go!

HEALING: NOT MANAGING

In my book, *The 10-Day Total Body Revolution*, I talk about how our minds and souls need to be altered to be able to *Revolutionize* our lives and the lives of everyone with whom we interact. I believe this is the key to sustained healing of our bodies.

I believe God can supernaturally heal us. If this does not happen for you, I believe God gives us wisdom to look to nature for our healing. All medicines are based on natural sources; they are just refined and altered into substances in a laboratory somewhere as some type of synthetic drug.

I tell people all the time, if you need to take a drug for a short amount of time then that is up to you; I assign no condemnation for so doing. HOWEVER, if you would like to try the natural approach then you will not have all the side effects of those drugs destroying many other parts of your body or causing you to have some other worse medical condition.

Natural therapies take longer for your body to use to correct damage than synthetic drugs that are formulated to go direct to the cause of problems.

Long term healing often takes a long-term approach. You must be willing to go the distance, fight the fight, and stay true to your course to achieve success. What that means is you develop a strategy and stay with it.

Do not divert to unhealthy foods or "forget" to take your supplements or to do your exercise routines. For rare, special occasions I will eat what I know is unhealthy, however I do not go ridiculously crazy in my eating. The cost is too great to "splurge" on a daily basis.

 Case in point, I love donuts, but they are killers! I will seldom now eat any type of pastry because they lead to cancers, high cholesterol, high blood pressure, and diabetes, Alzheimer's disease, heart disease and so much more. I know these truths as I am eating a packaged pastry item or a donut. That is why I eat them only rarely then I get back to my healthy lifestyle and work hard to counteract the ill effects of my divergent behaviour.

I discussed in the previous section how Pau d' arco helped kill Janie's tumour on her thyroid gland. Pau d' arco has been researched and tested and proven to kill tumorous cancer cells. Because cancer is so rampant in society I recommend it to everyone I know.

Olive Leaf Extract (OLE) is another herb I take on a daily basis and have been for a number of years. It is the leaves of the olive tree, pure and simple. This "extract" is a powder that has many benefits, but one of its keys is that it regulates our blood glucose. I have many testimonials of people who have suffered with diabetes and once they started taking OLE they have needed less and less of their medicine. A side effect of OLE is that it attacks belly fat; again there are numerous testimonials of people who have witnessed their body transformation once they started taking OLE.

I personally attest to the efficacy of St. John's Wort to bring my sleeping nerves back to life. I had back surgery years ago. My left leg was one half to two thirds numb. My leg felt like how you get a Novocain shot to deaden the pain for dental work, numb and useless. I walked with a limp and my doctor told Janie that I would eventually end up in a wheelchair if my nerves did not "wake up".

I would not settle for that type of prognosis. I researched natural cures for nerve pain and numbness and came across research for St. John's Wort that awakened sleeping nerves. I started taking the herb and before you know it I was walking straight again, not limping and even started jogging again.

These are just three products where we have realized healing and deliverance from pain and suffering. Everyone is different and I cannot claim they will work for you as they have for us and the people we know; however what if these products did work for you? Could your relief from pain and suffering be as close as taking a few supplements, altering your eating and drinking habits, changing your viewpoints on living and exercising differently?

CONCLUSION

This is what *Revolutionary Health* is all about! It is about shifting your belief patterns, using common sense, getting multiple medical opinions, trying different techniques or therapies and **NOT** giving up or giving in or saying I quit!

Fighters fight. Winners win. Overcomers overcome. If you have lost a battle, pick yourself up, get motivated and get going. Do not settle for someone else telling you how to live your life. Do not settle for some doctor or drug company trying to convince you that you need to take various pills for the rest of your life when all you have to do is alter your beliefs and practices and you could be living drug free.

Living drug free and being strong and healthy in my 60's I know I am truly blessed! Whatever your age, research the physical condition of the "average" person your age. Are you average? Do you take drugs on a regular basis whether that is prescription or over the counter medications? Do you consume the Standard American Diet (SAD)?

I have no plans on being "average", what about you? I will do whatever it takes to be strong and healthy. I will fight, not give up, never give in, continue to research foods, herbs and spices for their medicinal value and I never say die! Let's win this together!

CHAPTER 5

OVERWEIGHT NO MORE!
Part 1

You are in control of your life. Not your belly, not your cravings, not your addictions, not your past-nothing can control you to do that which you do not allow to be done to you if you do not allow it the opportunity to overcome you.

According to many medical journals, associations and governmental agencies, in 2018 over 70% of Americans are either overweight or obese. If you are a part of this statistic it is time you switched allegiances and lose the weight.

This chapter will focus specifically on addictions. The next chapter will state various strategies on how to fight obesity and being overweight.

ADDICTION FREE

We must get free from our addictions in order to live a healthy life. *Revolutionaries* are not addicts. We are not held captive to what friends, family, tradition or prior lifestyle dictates what we will eat and drink. We think for ourselves and willingly say NO to most foods and drinks.

Some clinics that try to help their patients get free from addictions, prescribe additional drugs. I understand that for some individuals this treatment program is successful, yet when we trade one drug for another the base root cause of the addiction may not be dealt with and needs attention. We need to be free from every type of addiction that can destroy our lives.

In this chapter we will first diagnose our addictions. You can describe it however you like: released from, delivered from, let go of or be free of our addictions; whatever it takes we must not be held captive by our food and drink addictions any longer.

First we must realize that we are addicts. There is no evil stereotype or connotations or condemnation implied with any term used in this book. To know if you are hooked on anything (food, drink, drug, lifestyle behaviour, mannerism, or anything else) we must first know what we are doing. This requires a diary.

Get out a pad of paper and pen right now and begin to write down everything, as much as you can remember, you have ate and drank today. Be as detailed as possible. Then go back to yesterday and do the same. Look in your refrigerator, freezer, and pantry or wherever you store your food and list out the basic quantities of types of foods you have. Think about the restaurants you frequent and types of food you consume.

List out how much meat, vegetables, fruit and starches you have in your home (not every single item, but a rough outline such as about five pounds of fruit). See how much pre-processed meals in boxes or bags you have stored. How much processed meat (sliced meat, bacon, sausage etc), processed cheese, and packages of cookies, chips, and crackers do you have? How many packaged beverages such as sodas, liquor, teas and juices do you have in your storehouse? Sweet pastries, deserts, ice cream, candy and the like; how much of sugar filled items do you have?

This is a chore, but it will help to open your eyes to what you are eating and drinking and to what you may be addicted. Now that you know what you HAVE, think about the volume of these items that you purchase on a regular basis.

Liquor kills brain cells, leads to Alzheimer's disease, increases risks of cancer, heart disease, diabetes, obesity, harms the liver and kidneys and is addictive. No one should drink any liquor of any type at any time. If you do consume any type of alcohol make it a point to decrease your consumption to eliminate it from your lifestyle completely as soon as possible.

Sweet drinks lead to obesity, cancers, Alzheimer's disease, heart problems and tooth decay. They lessen the natural body response to the "sweet" taste so we crave more sweets and they are extremely addictive. Sweetened drinks all need to be thrown out and never purchased again.

Processed foods: meats (salami, bologna, bacon, sausage etc.) are full of nitrates and cause cancer. Meals in packages, most types, are high in fats, sugar, and carbohydrates and "fake" food. I will talk more on "fake" food in the next chapter. Chips and crackers may taste great but those flavours you crave are fake and not real. These flavours are artificial chemicals that destroy your organs and lead to cancers, heart disease, obesity and more.

Dairy: there are natural chemicals in milk that make it addictive. Notice the innumerable types of cheese, yogurt and other types of dairy products that are available. Cheese is full of fat and preservatives and most yogurts have so much sugar that it is unbelievable; do your research. Cow's milk is for their calf, their baby; you are human and do not need the milk of a different mammal. Think about it.

This is just an overview of a few food types and how we must be set free from our addictions to them. Do you want to be free? Then follow these guidelines for your freedom from addiction.

Start with the worst offender in your home; let's say it is sweets. Throw out everything that is full of sugar from the list above and your inventory list. Stand in your kitchen and proclaim out loud:

"I want to be free from my addiction to sugar. I willingly make the choice today to rid my home of sugary foods and drinks. I admit that it is difficult for me not to eat and drink these things and I need help. I vow today, right now, right here to change my life.

"I do not want these foods and drinks to destroy my body or my mind anymore. I declare today that I am a *Revolutionary* and *Revolutionaries* are not addicted to anything. Every day I will be stronger in my resolve to be healthy and not eat and drink like I have in the past.

"I am worth it! I deserve to be healthy! I have lots to give to society and I want to be strong and healthy so I may live and not be sick or in pain. Right now, today I am free; I am delivered from my addiction to sugar."

How do you feel after saying that proclamation? You must do it out loud with authority and power for it to be effective. I have done this many times myself and with others and the effect is transformational!

Let's stay with the sugar addiction for a moment (you can use the above proclamation for any type of food, drink or behaviour and the following self analysis). Now, look back into your past and see if there is a reason you need "sugar" in your life. I do not mean the actual substance, but the emotion, the feeling of sweetness or love. Do you need the physiological aspects of "sugar" in your life?

Sugar addictions sometimes start by our need for love, family, attention and affection. This is why we crave to be "sweetened" by candy, pastry and similar products. Sometimes we must deal with this reason behind our actual food craving to be free from the actual addiction. This is real and affects most people who are addicted to sweets, whether they would admit to it or not.

If you were abused, neglected, molested, not wanted, abandoned or any other number of terrible conditions, we must be set free from the harmful emotions of rejection so we may not be addicted to sugar. Many people do not want to admit to this or do not understand this but those who embrace the need for freedom from harmful emotions and what I call "soul wounds" are the ones who are freed from their sugar addictions quicker and easier than those who do not embrace these beliefs.

This is real. I have released myself from harmful emotions from my past and have seen many people also set free through this technique of cutting soul ties. It is not easy to do; it is packed with emotions of pain and sorrow and with unbelief.

Many people do not believe they have a problem and adopt what I call the "tough guy" stance. They say to me, "I don't have a problem, I just like this kind of food and not you or anyone else is going to make me stop eating and drinking what I want!" That is their choice, however if they stay on the path they are on, sooner not later they will have a medical problem that makes them alter their lifestyle eating and drinking.

To break harmful soul ties we must let go, forgive and release those that hurt us in the past. It is not easy to be free from these ties on us; but when we release these soul-ties we can begin to live our new life. We live a *Revolutionary* life, not a fake life. Fake people are so easy to spot. Let us move from "fakery" to reality.

To release soul-ties, stand up, read and believe the following **<u>out loud</u>**:

"I release and break every soul-tie in my past. Everyone who has hurt me in any way I release his or her power over me. I will not give in to sorrow or despair any longer. I will not grieve over the past any longer. I forgive myself and I forgive anyone and everyone who harmed me.

"I am free from the destructive power of harmful emotions from my past. I pronounce and declare that I am a free person! I am unshackled from any bondage that previously held me back. I let go of the past and am able to live wonderfully today and for the rest of my life.

"I pronounce my freedom from all addictions. I no longer feel a need to overeat, or drink what harms my body and I accept myself. I love myself. I am a new person who can handle any situation in life without relying on food or drink to make it through the day. I am a new person! I am free! I am loved!"

Did you stand up and make your proclamation out loud? If not, get up and do that now. Repeat the proclamation over and over if you need to do so. That will only reinforce your determination and help you move forward in your new *Revolutionary* life. Make your proclamation out loud for the world to hear, even if you are alone somewhere. These kind of out loud, bold and forceful declarations have power and will transform you into the new person you want to be.

Making a verbal proclamation as the above may seem foolish, useless or a waste of time, yet believe me this type of "therapy", if you will believe it works. I believe with God's help you can accomplish what you determine to do and proclamations as these are the pathway towards your freedom from **ANY** type of addiction. Proclaim your freedom and walk in a new light of understanding from where you have come and to where you are going.

Now that you are free from addictions and soul-ties, let's take the next step in your *Revolutionary* walk.

<u>CONCLUSION</u>

Living addiction free is the life to live! When our soul-ties are broken from our past we can excel in everything we determine to accomplish. Making your personal pronouncements verbally can change your life in ways unimaginable.

Although we may be free from the "bondages" of various foods, drinks, painful past memories or traumatic events in our lives that does not mean that we will not have struggles. Through our vigilance in being observant of our mood swings, outside influences and tempting culinary delights we can stay in our *Revolutionary* mindset.

With the stumbling blocks of addictions and soul-ties severed we can move into a new realm, a *Revolutionary* realm where we conquer any "foe" in our path and achieve the lifestyle we want. Moving forward with our lives we now determine for ourselves a future no longer hindered by that which has held us back previously.

CHAPTER 6

OVERWEIGHT NO MORE!
Part 2

With each chapter you read you are becoming more and more informed on how to have *Revolutionary Health*. You realize it is *more* than just eating this or not eating that. It is more than drinking this or not drinking that. Your goal is to know who you are, who you <u>do not</u> want to be, who you **want** to be and to *become* everything that you are supposed to be.

Revolutionary Health is about you discovering the real you in this jaded, cynical, pretend, fake, artificial and mixed up world.

You have become motivated, you have decided to heal yourself and not be managed by others; you are free from addictions and soul ties so now you are ready to take your next *Revolutionary* steps.

It is time to review a broad array of aspects of the new you, the *Revolutionary* you.

FAKE, ARTIFICIAL OR REAL

You are not fake or artificial so it is time to stop eating, drinking, believing and living fake and artificial.

I am truthful in everything I do. I am tactful, but honest. I do not say or do things just to be accepted by various persons or groups of people. I seek to improve myself in every way that I can, but not so that I may please my peers. I am not a faker. Do fakers eat fake food? I am a real person therefore I prefer real food.

As a real person I want to eat real food every day for every meal, what about you? Once you set this standard, we must stick to our beliefs, insist upon pure food and drink and not fake food.

Let's start with what we drink. I drink at least one half my body weight in ounces of water or unsweet herbal tea daily. Most people can safely do this up to a gallon a day, depending on your weight. Include if you wish unsweetened herbal teas you brew your own; no store bought bottled tea any more whatsoever. I also drink home brewed coffee daily.

That is all we should drink, with a few exceptions. No sodas, alcohol, bottled juices, energy or sports drinks, or any other type of sweetened drink. The specialty coffees at various coffee houses are only for extremely rare occasions. Your body recognizes all of these drinks as harmful and wants their artificial, fake ingredients purged as soon as possible.

There are very few other beverages that would be acceptable, such as Kombucha, homemade juices and smoothes of whole foods-not fake ingredient powders, if you desire *Revolutionary Health*. Many stores now carry a wide variety of Kombucha, it is extremely healthy and you can make it yourself.

Discussing real food can take the rest of this book and additional volumes. I will give here a number of examples of the types of foods you should and should not eat. This quick review is so you will understand my point.

What you eat and drink should be that actual substance. The food should not be loaded with preservatives, artificial flavors, additives, sugars, salts or any other substance. We must learn or relearn how to prepare food at home. We must make the time to create healthy and wholesome food at home and not go out to eat all the time or have rushed, pre-packaged "food" that is harming us.

If you eat chips, which you should not, they should taste like the vegetable from which they were created, such as potatoes, corn, broccoli or cauliflower; any other flavour is artificial and harmful to your body. The same goes for crackers; think about it, these are made of flour, oil and salt, thus are naturally flavourless.

Vegetables and fruit are great fresh from the farmers market, frozen and pickled (in most cases) just watch for extra flavors or sugars that may be added. Any type of vegetable or fruit that has been processed or repackaged should probably be avoided; there are always exceptions but this is a general rule.

The only fats I suggest are olive oil, coconut oil and a little grapeseed oil. Depending on the diet or government source you follow, authors of scientific papers may expound the virtues of other fats. I like to keep things simple: foods less processed and to restrict the number and variety of fats. That is all our body needs; use common sense and balance when consuming fats in regards to cholesterol and various health issues you may be fighting. DO YOUR OWN RESEARCH.

MEAT AND SHELLFISH

If you eat meat, eat real meat, do not eat anything that has already been sliced, made into strips or pieces, processed, encased, or put into microwaveable containers. That is easy. Follow that basic rule as the first step in your "meat" *Healthy Revolution*. Yet, please, for your own health, cut WAY back on the volume of meat you consume, you are probably eating way too much for your actual bodily needs.

Processed meats include bacon and all the encased meats such as bologna, sausage, hot dogs, bratwurst and salami. Also included in this list of processed meats are the sliced meats at your market deli counter and available at sandwich shops; never ever eat these again! These are all loaded with artificial chemicals and preservatives and are the scrap, wasted parts of the animal that have been "mushed" together. They contain many types of seasonings added to be palatable and sold as speciality foods.

These processed meats are a prime cause of various types of cancers and heart disease. Avoid all these types of meats at all costs! If you already have intestinal problems, Crohns Disease, are overweight, kidney/gall bladder/liver problems or have been diagnosed with heart disease rid your home of these and never eat them again!

I do not advise eating any type of shellfish. I have never routinely eaten any type of shellfish and the last I had was back in the 1980's. Shellfish include clams, oysters, scallops, jellyfish, crayfish, shrimp, lobsters, crabs, mussels and similar sea creatures. These crustaceans are bottom feeders, meaning they eat all the dead junk on the bottom of the ocean and what is attached to ships or rocks or corals.

In some of the classes I took on safe food preparation, when Janie and I owned our restaurant and manufactured gourmet foods, I learned how unsafe shellfish were to consume. They are contaminated with numerous parasites and bacteria that we will ingest if they are not prepared properly to eat. The best way to avoid the numerous types of illnesses you can contract from eating these creatures, is simply do not eat them ever again!

HOME MEDICAL EQUIPMENT

During some of my teaching seminars I have listed a few inexpensive medical items or devices that I believe should be in every home; you probably already have some of the items. Invest in the equipment you do not have. Each item can have entire books written about their functions, how they track our health, guidelines on how to remain healthy when using these devices and innumerable other tips. The equipment listed here is for your introduction to a healthy lifestyle and to conduct your own further research of the devices and methods to improve your health.

You should use these on a regular basis to track your basic health. Observe your health first hand. If you come up unhealthy from any of these tests, follow more strenuously the guidelines within this book. Make immediate alterations to your lifestyle and get into your *Revolutionary Healthy* Zone.

1. **Thermometer.** Track your internal temperature. I have noticed that my temperature runs a little cool, less than 98.6 degrees. My extremities are often cool so I know I must be aware of any circulatory issues. Take your temperature on a regular basis.

2. **Digital Scale.** Track your weight. Do not become obsessed, but know your weight. Refer to a Body Mass Index scale, readily available on the Internet, and check your score. Using your scale and the BMI chart keeps you focused on being healthy and getting into the BMI healthy area-this is your *Revolutionary Healthy* Zone.

3. **pH Test Strips.** Available at most health foods stores. These little strips will show your body acidity or alkalinity, most of us are too acidic. You need to become pH balanced so you may strengthen your immune system and fight off diseases.

4. **Blood Pressure Cuff.** There are many varieties of these devises available at most pharmacy type stores. Big box discount stores may have a blood pressure measuring machine in their pharmacy department; avail yourself of this equipment. Monitor your blood pressure once a week. Make immediate small changes to your lifestyle as needed so a major health emergency will not surprise you. You should be in the range of 120/80.

5. **Blood Glucose Meter.** Pharmacy type stores carry a wide variety of these devices, test strips and lancets. Yes it hurts a little to draw your own blood, but you need to know what your blood glucose number is so you can track if you are becoming pre-diabetic. Most Americans are on track to become diabetic due to our extremely unhealthy eating habits. In an upcoming chapter there will be further discussion about optimum blood sugar levels.

6. **Blood Cholesterol Tests.** I am writing this book in late 2018 and have seen a few of these devises becoming available. As you are able to afford it, pick one up, and start tracking your numbers. There are many details to know regarding your blood cholesterol levels and I do not know the types of results these machines will give, but any information you get will be helpful. With this knowledge you can make healthy choices regarding your cholesterol levels.

This equipment is vital for you to have *Revolutionary Health*. By knowing your basic health numbers through the listed items you can make high quality decisions regarding your lifestyle eating and drinking habits and consider modifying your exercise routine.

DIET OR LIFESTYLE

There are an incredible number and variety of diets and weight loss programs available for you to follow. Some are good, some are bad and some are simply foolish or dangerous. Exercise equipment is readily available of any size, type and price range. Utilize common sense in regards to exercise equipment and "lifestyle" eating and drinking programs. Research the wide variety of scientific and medical studies on the exercise equipment and "lifestyle" you want to emulate and then go for it and change what needs to be changed.

For your *Revolutionary Health* and weight loss it is important to change what you need to change as soon as possible so you can do everything you need to do as quickly as you can. Small changes are easier to maintain, yet for the *Revolutionary*, make one **BIG** change and then work in smaller ones as you go.

For example: you completely give up drinking any type of alcohol and soda. This is a GIGANTIC change for some people. Another would be to walk for at least 45 minutes daily. Not just a casual stroll, but where you feel the burn in your legs and become out of breath. These are big changes for some people.

You are unique so you need a unique weight loss, muscle building, soul healing, and thought-changing program. Take the numerous ideas in this book; make a list of what you want to change ***FIRST*** and how you are going to change then start your one BIG change.

Do not pick a weight loss program, any program, and try to make it work, it will not. Remember all you learned in this chapter and the previous chapters, now let's jump into your new lifestyle.

CONCLUSION

In the next chapter we will go into detail about what foods and drinks to avoid and to consume on a regular basis. There is no reason why you cannot lose weight. By losing weight and eating correctly you will have less or no joint pain, back pain and digestive related conditions.

When in your *Revolutionary Healthy Zone*, pH balanced, and eating correctly you are less likely to contract colds and the yearly influenza virus, your risk for diabetes, various cancers, and heart disease and organ failures greatly diminishes. Your energy levels will go through the roof, you will feel and look younger and your skin will glow.

Your *Revolutionary* life is worth forbidding fast food, ice cream, fried junk food, sodas, liquor and pastries. Many, many people are waiting on you to become your REAL you, the strong you, the energetic you and now as a *Revolutionary* your time has come to shine!

CHAPTER 7

LET FOOD BE YOUR MEDICINE

Food can heal and it can kill. We will discover in short chapter divisions here how to eat healthy, what to eat and what not to eat. This chapter will be a launching pad for the next three chapters that will give specific information regarding wellness conditions that plague most people and how you can either avoid them or get stronger and healthier if you suffer from them.

There are many factors that play into our health: genetics, location where we live, environmental issues, soul-wounds, stubbornness (good and bad), current medical condition and vision for the future. When we develop the mentality of the first three chapters: NEVER GIVE UP, NEVER GIVE IN, and NEVER SAY DIE we open ourselves to great possibilities of healing and being inspirational to others.

Jump into the subsections of this chapter with an open heart and determination to change and you will see amazing results.

<u>WATER</u>

Drink water, as I mentioned in Chapter 6, to begin your detoxification process. Water is your first and best way to cleanse your system and to get your body in balance.

Most people can safely drink up to one half their body weight in ounces of water and unsweet herbal tea. Do not go over one gallon of fluids, this may be too much depending on your weight.

Water flushes our kidneys, helps with our digestion, is nourishing to our skin, aides in the distribution of nutrients throughout our system and keeps us hydrated. Increase your water and possibly unsweet herbal tea intake and decrease any other drink that is harmful to your body.

I routinely drink nearly a gallon of water and tea daily and seem to have boundless energy. Yes, I need to use the restroom often, but I purge out my morning coffee through drinking water and any toxins that may build up in my kidneys and liver.

When you go out to eat, drink only water with citrus or unsweet tea, nothing else. Graduate up to unsweet tea no longer using any type of sweetener if all you drink is sweet tea. Develop a "taste" for water and unsweet tea and your body will thank you.

STRETCHING

I lay with my back flat on the floor, legs up and over my navel. I stretch my back like this almost every morning. I sometimes hold a weight as I stretch my back. During this time I also stretch my arms over my head and out sideways as far as I can reach. While doing these movements I can feel my back shift and move into place and relieve any pressure there may be in my bones or joints.

Get going with stretching your arms and legs. Twist around, lift your arms high, step high, do squats (hold onto a chair at first if you need for balance) and get your joints all limbered up. Then get out and start moving. If you sit all day, get up to stretch your legs and move your body at least every 15 minutes.

Have you heard the phrase motion is lotion to your joints? If you sit still you will stiffen up and not be able to do what you need to do and will complain about joints that hurt or "pop". So, get up, get going, stretch and get your body moving.

For details on specific stretching exercises you can go online and study many types of routines. You can also reference my book *The 10-Day Total Body Revolution* for more ideas on stretching.

GROUNDING OR EARTHING

I heard about this concept back in 2015 and have been purposefully doing it ever since. Little did I know, but Janie has been "grounding" since she was a child. Ever since Janie was young she has been running around outside barefoot.

Grounding or earthing is going barefoot on the ground (earth, rocks, sand and soil). Your body will receive the electromagnetic energy that passes through the earth, into your bare feet and help align your body.

There are many scientific research papers, alternative medicine doctor reports and qualified persons who practice this on a regular basis. Do your own research on this subject and see what you think.

I like to go outside early in the morning, take a cup of coffee and stand around on the grass in front of our house while watching the sunrise. It is quiet where I live and peaceful so I am able to get myself grounded.

I am able to think clearly and pray to God while looking up at the gradually lightening sky, as the stars slowly disappear from sight. I get my thoughts together for the day ahead and feel at peace with my surroundings. Get out there and get grounded.

GOOD FATS

My morning routine begins as I chop up two cloves of garlic and take them with a little raw, organic honey and a half a glass of water. I start a small pot of weak coffee then stretch on the floor for ten minutes get my cup of coffee and go outside to get grounded.

When I make my cup of coffee I use a teaspoon of coconut oil. The good saturated fat of coconut oil feeds my brain and is the only saturated fat I consume.

I like using olive oil, grapeseed oil and coconut oil. Some diets call for a large daily intake of these or other oils/fats but I prefer only a small amount daily. Due to the fact that I do not eat greasy fried foods or "prepared meals", store bought cookies or other foods that contain transfats or saturated fats I consume a correct balance of good fats.

We need fat in our lifestyle eating and these are the preferred ones. As we consume less bad fats (meat, deep fried foods, chips, cookies, crackers etc) we need the balance of these good fats to "feed" our brain the nutrition it needs. Two tablespoons of good fats daily are enough for most people.

Enjoy other good fats such as avocado and flax along with chia seeds. There are others, but stick with these to be *Revolutionary*. There is no need to stock your pantry with all types of oils and fats; use these few on a daily basis and you will enjoy great health. Remember common sense and balance when using fats, but do not be afraid of them you need the RIGHT fat in your life.

EXERCISE

Now that you have had your morning garlic with water, coffee (if you drink it) with coconut oil, stretched and grounded it is time to exercise.

Exercise whenever, wherever, however you can. Work up to it, but push yourself to your limit, see how much you can do and then do more. It is not until we push ourselves, in every aspect of our lives, that we discover our full potential.

If you have never exercised before, this is your AHA moment when you realize, this is it-this is the time I begin to get healthy. Walk, jog, get on your treadmill or elliptical machine and get going. Get out the free weights and start pumping iron. All the equipment in the world is no good if you do not use it.

Some fitness centers charge only $10.00 per month to join and use their facilities. Make the time, get in there, talk to a trainer and start a routine that will build up your stamina and muscles. You need strong muscles, limber joints and less of a belly (and everywhere else that collects fat).

Through exercise you reduce stress, increase your lung capacity, detox through sweat, increase your digestive capabilities, lose weight, escalate your endurance and strengthen your immune system.

Remember, this is not just some diet book or some book by a motivational speaker or a book of nice and safe suggestions-this is a book that seeks to radically transform you into a person with *Revolutionary Health!* The only way to have *Revolutionary Health* is to do *Revolutionary* acts that stem from *Revolutionary* beliefs.

So I challenge you to challenge yourself to get healthy through believing differently, eating and drinking differently, exercising differently and looking at yourself differently. Join that fitness center, buy the equipment you need and make room for it at home and get out there in the heat, the cold, the rain and the wind and push you to excellence!

GOOD EATS

Eat food that feeds and nourishes your body, not "food" that inflames, feeds fungus and cancers, blocks your arteries and raises your blood glucose level, your blood pressure and cholesterol. It is possible to eat to become and stay healthy. You have to be *Revolutionary* according to most people, but that is what you are; you are unique and past ready for a change in your life.

In the next subsection I will describe foods and drinks to decrease or eliminate from your life where you will be saving LOTS of money so you can now afford to eat healthy.

Your new life will center on the produce section of your local grocery store. Fresh raw produce and fresh and dried herbs and spices will be the new staple in your life. The rest of the grocery store will have very little in it that you will want as you progress in your *Revolutionary* life.

You should be eating a couple of big handfuls of leafy greens daily. I take a small container of greens to work with me often to munch on as a snack. Put a big handful in a skillet on low heat with a little water in the pan. Let the greens warm and wilt slightly, dash with powdered garlic and enjoy. Salads, stir-fry, fresh for snacks-however you want them eat them, but just do it every day.

Spinach, kale, collards/turnip/beet/mustard greens, Romaine, red and green leaf lettuces, broccoli, Swiss chard, red cabbage, Bok Choy, parsley, arugula, buttercrisp, Bibb, and many other types of loose leaf "greens" are available for you to enjoy.

Make a green smoothie for breakfast or an evening meal. Start with a huge handful of any of the above greens, add a couple of ounces if you like of coconut or almond milk, a tablespoon of coconut oil, ice and one green apple. From there you can change it up by adding a stalk or two of celery, a small zucchini squash, an avocado and/or a few slices of cucumber.

Carrots, sweet potatoes, butternut squash, peppers, tomatoes, various onions, beets, radishes, rhubarb, apples, strawberries, grapes, cranberries, grapefruit, pomegranates and watermelon are a few of your red and orange vegetables and fruit. You need some of each of these daily to have a balanced lifestyle. Sauté, stir fry, raw in salads, smoothies, baked, tossed into stews and soups and fresh and raw as snacks are some of the ways to fix these vegetables and fruit.

There are many other vegetables to choose from, these are only a small sampling. Vegetables should be at least half of everything you eat every day. Two fruit a day is fine, a few ounces of protein and some complex carbohydrates will round out your daily routine.

I recommend very little if any animal protein; look back at chapter 6 on meat and shellfish. I eat an extremely small amount of beef, chicken or fish and no pork or shellfish. I prefer to get the bulk of my protein through beans, seeds, nuts and various grains. A cup of cooked beans, some nuts, a big scoop of quinoa, amaranth, millet or _many_ other psudograins drizzled with olive oil and a few dashes of powdered garlic and I have all the protein I need. Research non-meat sources of protein and you will be surprised.

Vegetable and grain carbohydrates as mentioned will keep you fit, full and healthy. Pasta, breads, tortillas, white rice, potatoes and other starches turn to sugar in our body so too much of these is very unhealthy. Strive for smaller amounts of quality rather than large amounts of bulk, for example have a cup of quinoa instead of burger buns and bread at restaurants.

Fill yourself daily with the good eats-lots of vegetables, plenty of leafy greens, two pieces of fresh fruit, a little quality protein and healthy fat with some whole grains. You will be losing weight and getting stronger every day following this routine.

<u>BAD EATS</u>

I will not belabor the points here, we all know what we should not eat, but I will spell it out for you. If you want to be a *Revolutionary*, if you want *Revolutionary Health* and if you determine to rid your life of the following foods you will become strong, healthy, disease resistant and be the leader, the example to your world that people need to follow and emulate.

Sugar: it is in sweet drinks, pastries and nearly every processed food product in the grocery stores. Cancer, heart disease and diabetes get worse the more you consume sweet foods and drinks. Remember how to free yourself from your sugar addiction (chapter 5), most all of us have a problem with too much sugar. Free yourself of this deadly substance and you will live longer and healthier.

Salt: we need a little of it in our lives, but very little. It is a preservative used in all packaged and canned foods. Eliminate these types of products, hide the saltshaker and use just a pinch and your heart will thank you.

Cheese: is high in fat, is a leading cause of high cholesterol, and is seemingly slathered on everything and anything served in a restaurant. Americans are drowning in their cheese addictions. Casein is a protein found in all milk products that during digestion releases opiates called casomorphins, which trigger our dopamine receptors that release an addictive element into our bodies. If you are addicted to cheese admit it, become free from your addiction and live a life "cheese free".

Alcohol, tobacco and artificial sweeteners and flavors-do not consume any of these products any more. Artificial sweeteners and flavors are in most packaged and processed food so much that these toxins have been accepted by most people. To *Revolutionize* your life choose daily more and more fresh, real, whole foods rather than packaged or "premade" meals of any type.

Alcohol and tobacco will kill you. They have no nutritional value, inflame the body lead to a myriad of diseases including numerous cancers, Alzheimer's Disease, diabetes, heart disease, liver failure, kidney damage, digestive problems and many other conditions. No one should ever consume either of these products at any time if they desire to become healthy.

It takes more time and energy to cook real food than the fake, boxed, preprepared junk foods that are available, but you will live a stronger, healthier, disease free life if you choose to live in this manner.

Deep-fried foods and fast foods which are heavy on the bad oils, salt and starchy carbohydrates (breads, potato products, rice, chips and the like) kill people every day through obesity, cancers, heart disease, kidney failure and gall bladder problems. It is EASY to avoid these illnesses by simply choosing to eat differently, thinking about a long healthy future (not a quick hunger fix) and caring for your body through a right mind rather than allowing an addicted body overrule your brain.

CONCLUSION

Change your lifestyle, not your diet. Live a new life.

Plan and prepare for a long and healthy future by making quality decisions today. Do not allow your stomach to control your life, use your brain and heart.

Decide on motivational factors that will propel you towards a healthy future where you lead people through your *Revolutionary* lifestyle rather than you being led by the nose by people whose goal is to take money from you with their pills, potions, portion controlled foods, drinks and gadgets.

Take one big step followed by small steps that you have fashioned into goals that you can keep and are manageable.

You are in control of your life. Do not allow people to guilt trip you, manipulate you, con or push you into doing what you know is not right.

Make losing weight and being healthy a directive, a prerogative in your life.

Eat more foods earlier in the day and less as the day progresses.

Plan and prepare healthy snacks having them available as you need and want them throughout the day.

Discover the new, healthy you and live a *Revolutionary* life.

CHAPTER 8

REVOLUTIONIZE CANCER

There are many books, research studies, and blogs, traditional and alternative therapies by which a person may research cancer. The topic is inflammatory to many due to how cancer has affected their life or the lives of loved ones.

This short chapter is by far non-inclusive of all research, statistical evidence or practices related to the prevention and treatment of cancer. I will share a few points and *Revolutionary* practices for you to ponder upon and decide for yourself.

I acknowledge that no one plan of action seems to be a cure or preventative practice that will insure a person from contracting any form of cancer. My hope is that through enacting multiple strategies we can lessen our risk factors, increase our immunity and strengthen our resolve to fight cancer with every ounce of strength and particle of determination that we have available to us.

HISTORY OF CANCER

The disease was first called cancer by the ancient Greek physician Hippocrates (460-370 BC). He is considered the "Father of Medicine." Hippocrates used the terms carcinos and carcinoma to describe non-ulcer forming and ulcer-forming tumors. In Greek these terms mean "a crab". The description was because the finger like spreading projections from a cancer called to mind the shape of a crab.

From ancient to modern times, doctors have theorized how cancer cells develop in the body. Doctors and researchers continue to consider reasons as to why some people contract this illness. Various tests and screenings have been developed over the years, yet none of these aid the patient on how to **AVOID** or **PREVENT** cancers from developing in the first place.

Surgery, radiation therapy, chemotherapy, and immunotherapy have been developed to try to destroy cancers that grow in the body. Cancer cells originate from normal cells when the DNA within the cell nucleus is damaged. Our DNA sometimes becomes mutated when our cells divide. Cell division occurs constantly throughout our lives and often mutations will happen to them.

Mutations in our cells occur due to tobacco smoke, radiation, and ultraviolet radiation from the sun, artificial substances in our foods (sweeteners, additives and flavors) and chemicals in our environment. Carcinogenic compounds in foods or food processing mutate the DNA within our cells that lead to cancer.

Additives in foods and drinks that are carcinogenic (mutate our cells into becoming cancerous) are substances that are used to prolong shelf life, storage life, enhance color, flavor and texture. Other substances include growth hormones in animal food, antibiotics, pesticides and herbicides and heavy metals such as cadmium and mercury.

Processed meats such as lunchmeat, ham, hot dogs and other encased meats and other such foods have nitrites added during the manufacturing process, which causes mutation of our DNA and can lead to various types of cancer. **SO STOP EATING ANY OF THEM!**

There are many types of cancers that occur that doctors have no explanation as to why the person's cells mutated as such to cause cancer. In these cases research is ongoing to find a cause then a treatment to keep the cancer from developing in the first place.

CANCER RISK FACTORS AND PREVENTION

A number of types of cancers cannot be attributable to a single cause, yet for those that can the risk factors may be divided into four distinct groups:

1.   Biological or internal factors such as age, gender, inherited genetic defects and skin type.

2.   Environmental exposure such as radon and UV radiation and fine particulate matter.

3.   Occupational risk factors include working amid carcinogenic chemicals, radioactive materials and asbestos.

4.   Lifestyle related factors.

This section will focus on the lifestyle-related factors that we may be able to control. It has been well researched and documented that tobacco, alcohol, UV radiation from sunlight and nitrites and poly aromatic hydrocarbons generated by barbecuing foods are cancer causing factors we can control and limit.

Through the elimination from our lifestyle: tobacco, alcohol, barbecued and smoked foods, processed meats (as described in the prior section) and packaged foods that contain artificial flavors, colors, textures and chemicals to preserve and prolong shelf life we can **_GREATLY_** reduce the risk of developing cancer.

Through review of products that are contaminated with heavy metals we can also eliminate another avenue of cancerous mutation of our DNA. This would include the elimination of most if not all seafood from our eating. Heavy metal contamination of seafood is well known and documented.

We should analyse the types of make up, creams, lotions and deodorant products that are used which may contain heavy metals. Beast cancer, in some cases, may be linked to heavy metals in deodorant products.

Revolutionaries-if you have not heard this information before, you are responsible for it now. To reduce the risk of getting cancer it is imperative to alter your lifestyle eating and drinking habits IMMEDIATELY and due further personal research.

<u>**ALTERNATIVE MEDICAL THERAPIES**</u>

Throughout my life I have eaten nearly every type of cancer causing food and drank nearly every type of cancer causing drink. So what can I do about it now? Is it too late for me? Am I doomed to get cancer?

A loud and resounding <u>***NO***</u> is the answer to the above questions! Your first step is to clear out your food and drink pantry, refrigerator and freezer of any and all cancer causing agents. Second do not buy them anymore or order them at restaurants.

Now let's clean up our bodies and fight what cancer may be growing. Remember in Chapter 4 Healing Not Managing and the subsection on Paradigm Shifting when I shared about Janie and her thyroid problems. We both take the herb Pau'd arco daily to fight any type of tumor growth in our bodies. We take between 1,000-2,000 milligrams daily. I list our herbal/spice source in the Bibliography and References section of this book (I receive no remuneration from this recommendation).

Detox your home of heavy metal cleaning agents. Aluminium in your cookware will leech into the foods you prepare; be aware of the same problem with cast iron skillets.

Internal detoxification of your kidneys, liver, intestines and gall bladder are important. These are the filtering and cleansing agents in your body. If they are clogged up with toxic materials, then you will suffer from a fatty liver, diverticulitis, kidney and gallstones, leaky gut syndrome and many other conditions.

The following are natural detoxifiers that aid our bodies in fighting cancer by cleansing toxins from our system. Turmeric kills cancer cells and stops them from spreading. Sage helps to fight cancer and improves our memory. Besides fighting cancer Cumin boosts our immune system and helps to regulate our blood glucose levels. Cinnamon, use it in your coffee and oatmeal; it fights cancer. Cayenne pepper is effective in fighting many types of cancers.

Garlic is a great natural detoxifying anti-cancer agent. I cut up two cloves of garlic the first thing every morning and take it with a little honey. I use garlic in nearly every dish I cook. I use ginger, black pepper, oregano and rosemary daily in my battle to fight cancer.

If you will start incorporating these practices and begin cooking with herbs you will be fighting the battle against cancer. There are many other practices you can do by doing your own research; for the *Revolutionary* these are great beginning steps to take in your war strategy.

SUGAR AND CANCER

Is there a connection between sugar and cancer?

The American Institute for Cancer Research states on their website that "There is no strong evidence that directly links sugar to increased cancer risk, yet there is an indirect link."

All cells, including cancerous cells, need sugar from our bloodstream for fuel. If we would cut down on the amount of sugar in our bloodstream cancer cells would not be able to receive the fuel they need to survive.

The fact that cancer cells need sugar to grow stands to reason that if we cut back and could nearly eliminate it and refined carbohydrates such as white flour, high fructose corn syrup, sodas and other sweetened beverages from our lifestyle we can stop feeding tumors and cancer growth.

Cancer cells uptake sugar at 10-12 times the rate of healthy cells. PET scans routinely use radioactively labelled glucose to detect sugar hungry tumor cells.

In 1931 Otto Warburg, PhD Nobel laureate in medicine discovered that cancer cells have a different energy metabolism than healthy cells. He found that tumors used glucose as fuel at a faster rate than healthy cells.

Cancer thrives in an acidic environment, sugar is acidic and most of us have highly acidic metabolisms. Sugar suppresses our immune system making it harder for our bodies to fight off cancerous tumors. A four-year study at the National Institute of Public Health and Environmental Protection in the Netherlands discovered that sugar intake was associated with more than double the risk for breast cancer in women.

Sugar is known to be a cause for being overweight and obese which in turn is a high risk factor for developing various types of cancers, such as esophageal, pancreatic, kidney, breast, gallbladder and colorectal.

CONCLUSION

REVOLUTIONARIES-to effectively fight cancer it is time to end our addiction to sugar, lose weight, exercise, get free from soul-wounds, stop eating bacon and hot dogs, no more smoked or barbequed foods and start eating pure, whole foods.

Start today improving your health, lessening your risk factors for cancer and get out there and live the life of a leader, a person who thinks for her and himself, is not pressured to eat and drink like everyone else and is a *REVOLUTIONARY* in all aspects of life!

CHAPTER 9

REVOLUTIONIZE HEART DISEASE

Heart disease is responsible for one in four deaths in the United States every year. Do not become a statistic. Become a *Revolutionary* and do not join the growing number of people who have heart disease.

To be a *Revolutionary*, you must think different, you must act different and you must become a different person. This is not impossible; it is very easy if you have the means, the motive and the opportunity.

Revolutionaries change their circumstances; they do not allow circumstances to change them. It is time to act, react if you must if you are in poor health but act **NOW**!

Whether your means (financial situation) is strong or weak, start lifestyle changes immediately whatever you can afford to do, no excuses. Make as big of changes as you can afford and continually increase these changes.

Get motivated to not have heart disease. I tell people all the time you need to have a motivational factor to become a *Revolutionary,* in this case **<u>NOT</u>** to have heart disease. One of my motivational factors is to have a home on the beach somewhere when I retire and spend many years with Janie enjoying the beach.

I stated another motivational factor when my first grandson was born: "When my grandson's child graduates from college I want to be as healthy then as I am today". My grandson was born when I was 55 years old; I was in great shape then and am in even better physical condition today.

To have the opportunity to not have heart disease is as easy as determining in your soul that you will permanently alter your beliefs about eating and drinking and life in general. You are taking your opportunities to educate yourself by reading this book; now be sure to enact all the admonitions and suggestions to have *Revolutionary Health.*

<u>HERE'S YOUR SIGN</u>

Symptoms of a heart attack for women are some type of pain or discomfort in the chest, but are more than likely to have symptoms unrelated to chest pain such as neck, jaw, shoulder, upper back or abdominal pain, shortness of breath, pain in one or both arms, nausea or vomiting, sweating, lightheadedness or dizziness and unusual fatigue.

Major risk factors or causes for women to have heart disease are diabetes, mental stress and depression, tobacco use, inactivity, menopause, some drugs used to treat breast cancer, and complications during pregnancy.

Symptoms of a heart attack for men are chest discomfort (pain, tightness or pressure), nausea, indigestion, heartburn, stomach pain, pain that spreads to the left arm and left side of the body, feeling dizzy or lightheaded, throat or jaw pain, becoming exhausted, breaking out in a cold sweat and a cough that will not quit.

Major risk factors or causes for men to have heart disease include being age 45 or older, tobacco use, high blood pressure/cholesterol/blood glucose, being overweight, diabetes, lack of physical activity and stress.

As a *Revolutionary* I am often blunt and to the point. Let's get serious about <u>*preventing*</u> heart disease rather than reacting to it after the fact and having to take a fist full of pharmacological agents that will destroy our organs or have some type of surgical procedure.

Revolutionary methods to avoid a heart attack:

- Stop drinking any type of alcohol.

- Stop all tobacco use.

- Lose weight if you are overweight.

- End your sugar addiction.

- Get moving and exercise.

- Eat more vegetables than meat and potatoes.

- Completely stop eating red meat.

- Reduce to eliminate cheese consumption.

- No more deep-fried fast foods.

* No encased meats (hot dogs, sausage, salami) and all similar processed meats.

- Reduce stress.

We can end heart disease today, or at least greatly reduce it, if we would actually enact the above **Radical** *Revolutionary* concepts. These choices are **Radical** and *Revolutionary* because most people are stubborn and simply will not eat their greens and will not stop eating beef (there is much more to it than that to end heart disease, but you understand what I am saying).

Review each of these *Revolutionary* practices and see how they can be applied to your lifestyle. This is reiterating some material, but it is important to drive these points down into the depths of your being so you make them your new *Revolutionary* lifestyle.

Stop drinking any type of alcohol.

-Alcohol use destroys the liver, raises blood glucose levels, is a risk factor for cancer and heart disease, has **no** nutritional value, damages the kidneys and is a factor in weight gain. Stop all alcohol consumption immediately.

Stop all tobacco use.

-Tobacco contains dozens of toxins that are harmful to our bodies, is highly addictive, is not "cool", destroys our immune system, leads to various cancers and heart disease, is dirty, makes you stink and pollutes the environment. Stop using any and all tobacco products immediately.

Lose weight if you are overweight.

-You must do what it takes to get in shape, lose weight and be healthy. Join a fitness center. Join an organization that tracks your weight and gives meal preparation and fitness tips at weekly meetings. Your future, the future of your family, your business and interpersonal relationships depend on you getting in great physical condition. Start today!

End your sugar addiction.

-Admit you have a problem with sugar and overcome this addiction. You are stronger than ANY addiction! You are not identified by the way you look or behave as a sugar addict so now believe it and walk in your new identity. You do not need "sugar" psychologically or physically to cope with emotional problems. You have overcome all painful emotions therefore you are not bound to desiring sugar in any of its forms. You are a *Revolutionary* and you are free!

Get moving and exercise.

-Reference the Bonus Material at the end of this book. See Chapter 3 Exercise: Stretching, Aerobic, Anaerobic & HITT from my book *The 10-Day Total Body Revolution.*

Eat more vegetables than meat and potatoes.

-Eat more colorful foods and less meat. Colorful foods include salad greens, cruciferous vegetables (cabbage, broccoli, Brussel sprouts, Bok Choy and others), peppers, tomatoes, sweet potatoes, carrots and so many more (see the Good Eats subsection of Chapter 7 Let Food Be Your Medicine). At some point in the future there will be a "meat tax" enacted (like the 'sin tax' imposed on alcohol and tobacco products), so learn now to eat less and less meat, if for no other reason than to save money.

Completely stop eating red meat.

-Red meat is a killer, literally, when considering heart disease. Reduce to eliminate beef from your lifestyle as quickly as possible. You do not NEED it to live regardless of what you think and it will shorten your life. Even the grass fed, organic varieties; it is still beef and will cause damage to your organs and arteries. Just say no to beef and stop eating it!

Reduce to eliminate cheese consumption.

-Cheese is addictive, there are endless varieties of the stuff, and it is EVERYWHERE and on nearly everything that everyone eats! You do not need cheese. Regardless how much you like it, it does not like you. Milk is for baby cows; you are not a baby cow. Strive to reduce and eventually eliminate cheese from your lifestyle.

No more deep-fried fast foods.

-This is the bottom line: no more deep-fried fast foods. PERIOD!

If you do not want to have a stroke, heart attack, accelerate your blood pressure or cholesterol you will stop eating fried and deep fried foods at home or any type of restaurant. Do not deep-fry turkeys, catfish, corn fritters or anything else. The oils used to cook these foods in restaurants and at home (for most people), are some of the worst for your heart. Learn to see these foods as they really are-**DEATH**-so that you will not want them anymore.

It is not worth your life to pick up these foods when you can have a heart attack because of them. Fried chicken is loved by millions of people, yet is it worth dying for? I have had relatives who would not stop eating these foods and died from a heart attack; do not allow this to be your legacy.

No encased meats (hot dogs, sausage, salami) and all similar processed meats.

-I grew up eating all these kinds of meats, and loved them, but slowly over the years with my increased awareness on how unhealthy they are I have decreased to eliminate them from my life. I have eaten my weight many times over of sliced deli meats, bologna, sausage, hot dogs and the like so I only have myself to blame for any high blood pressure and cholesterol I have.

These are the true "junk meat" in the meat aisle of your grocery store. The artificial flavors, smoke, texturing agents and fillers are killers. These products are the by-products of animals that are not suitable for individual packaging so they are ground up and put in sausage, hot dogs, bratwurst, bologna, salami, pastrami and all other similar products. Stop the madness and stop eating these disgusting "meats".

Reduce stress.

-There are innumerable techniques to reduce stress. Go outside and breathe fresh air, go for a walk, stretch, join a book reading club, join a fitness center, talk with friends on social media, stand barefoot on the grass, watch the ocean waves crash onto the shoreline, take a hike in the mountains, the list goes on and on. Do not take pills or drink alcohol or eat junk or snack foods to reduce your stress; these actions only make your stress worse. Seriously, learn deep breathing techniques and walk around your house to get your circulation moving; you can reduce stress, you need to reduce stress to lessen the effects of heart disease.

<u>CONCLUSION</u>

Heart disease does not have to be the outcome for 25% or more of the population. You can make quality and quantitative changes in your life today, right now by enacting the *Revolutionary* techniques described in this chapter.

Sure, you may have heard it all before, none of this is new to you; however YOU are a new person in the reading of this book and YOU will not settle for the same old life you used to live.

You are in the middle of a metamorphisis. You are changing into a new person and that new person will not be afflicted by heart disease because you do not have any of the risk factors. You have already changed your life and are making daily alterations to what you believe and how you act that propel you into *Revolutionary Health*.

Be the leader, be the game-changer, be the one to whom everyone looks for answers when it comes to overcoming heart disease. Be the *Revolutionary* <u>they</u> need to move <u>them</u> into a new healthy lifestyle.

Your actions influence those with whom you associate. You can say anything you want, but your actions are what people notice. How you eat and drink. What you believe and do. Where you go to eat. Become the *Revolutionary* that has changed and does not practice the same old habits so those around you will want to become like you.

Soon people will be coming to you asking you what you have done to change your life and if they do what you have done can they look like you? Can they become as healthy as you? It will happen, believe me. So start transforming your life today, fight heart disease and be the living example of a *Revolutionary*!

CHAPTER 10

REVOLUTIONIZE

DIABETES

Diabetes does not have to be inevitable and incurable. It is not a normal condition that most people will contract. Prediabetes and type II diabetes can be easily avoided. Even though a relative has type II diabetes does not mean you will contract the illness.

Do those statements help dispel some fears that may have developed in you? Everyone can say they know a family member or friend who has or had cancer, heart disease or diabetes. That trend can change! That trend WILL change if we follow the advice of this book.

Do not settle for the curse that someone speaks over you that you are doomed to get cancer or have heart disease or become diabetic. Unfortunate and unforeseen things happen in our lives, yes, sometimes that includes these conditions, however that is not definite for any of us and we can fight against any and all diseases!

As of October 2018 the population of the United States is a little under 329 million people. Of that number, 3 million people have type I diabetes, 24 million have type II diabetes and 86 million have prediabetes. These numbers will skyrocket in the years to come because at least 70% or 230,000,000 of the total US population are overweight, many of whom do not control their blood glucose levels (the Centers for Disease Control and Prevention-CDC-reports that over 70% of Americans are overweight or obese).

Being overweight or obese does not cause Type II Diabetes, but is a risk factor and one reason why people become type II diabetic.

A blood glucose meter, available almost anywhere, measures the sugar level in our blood. Current medical research indicates that a fasting blood glucose level of 100 or *lower* is <u>normal</u>. A reading of 100-125 is prediabetic and a level over 125 is diabetic.

Revolutionaries do not back down, they do not give up, they do not give in, they do not say die. *Revolutionaries* are victorious because **they** change life situations that surround them-they are not changed *by* them.

TYPE I DIABETES

Type I diabetes is the inherited form of this condition and is usually diagnosed when a person is a child. In the past people did not know they had type I diabetes as a child and it suddenly came upon them as a young adult. The fear of this occurring has led many people to believe anyone at anytime can contract diabetes for no apparent reason.

Type I diabetes is genetic and affects a small number of the population. In the past, a person diagnosed with type I diabetes had nerve problems, vision problems, kidney disease and heart disease early in life and often died young. Today, when the disease is discovered early in a patient's life with proper medication and the strict adherence to proper nutrition the person is believed to have a normal life expectancy.

My father did not know he had diabetes until he was in his early 30's. He was apparently strong and healthy, but was slowly getting weaker due to the condition and then suddenly his whole life changed. He lived for approximately 20 years after his diagnosis; the last 10 years were full of pain and an ongoing further debilitating physical condition.

My father did not cause the disease to come upon him; it was beyond his control. These things happen to many people for many types of conditions. To me, reasons are inconsequential, something has happened now let's see what we can do about it.

If you or someone you know has type I diabetes do not play games with your insulin pump. I know people who eat and drink whatever they want and just allow their pump to put more insulin into their body. This disease destroys us organ by organ, leaving us in extreme pain and suffering if we do not *Revolutionize* our lifestyle.

<u>PREDIABETES</u>

Most people with prediabetes do not know they have elevated blood glucose levels. I advise everyone I meet and those whom I counsel to get their fasting blood glucose levels checked, and checked on a regular basis. When you know your number then you can make adjustments to your lifestyle.

Most of us are addicted to sugar and I know I am. Although I do not eat much sweetened foods or drinks, I know once I start it is hard to stop. One mini donut or candy bar turns into four. To be sure we do not contract this terrible illness, or heart disease or cancer we must be diligent, utilize self-control and stop consuming all the sweets that we do. We are literally eating ourselves to death!

In the summer of 2018 I went to a clinic to have my cholesterol and blood glucose levels checked. .

I found out a few days later, my fasting blood glucose reading that morning was 68. It was a little low because I had not eaten that morning, it should be low for that very reason. We want to strive to have our fasting blood glucose, checked first thing in the morning before we consume anything, to be 85 or under (**without** taking **any** medication).

Even though I have consumed sugar rich foods and drinks all my life, I have not gorged myself on them. Since the mid 1990's I have slowly consumed less and less sugary substances, yet especially since 2012 I have greatly cut back on these foods. Yes, I still do have some pastries or chocolates, yet it is much less often and I try to limit my intake. I must be doing something right because my number is always way under 100.

I do not take any medications for any illness, but do eat lots of garlic and take Olive Leaf Extract. Both of these are excellent for balancing my blood glucose levels and helping my body stay in balance.

You know my morning routine of garlic and honey; well I also usually take about 2,000 milligrams of Olive Leaf Extract daily (it is available in any health foods store or see the Selected Bibliography and References at the end of this book for my source).

Exercise, balanced eating, no sweet drinks, stress reduction techniques and soul healing have been keys to my maintaining low blood glucose numbers.

The **REAL** number of Americans with Prediabetes is MUCH MUCH higher than the medical community reports. The number of overweight Americans shows the trend towards diabetes.

Do not allow prediabetes to creep up on you and then before you know it you have full-blown type II diabetes. This is nothing to laugh off or disregard or discount or not take seriously. You do not have to be a victim of this or any other illness, but you must take your health seriously.

To truly live we all **must** become *Revolutionaries.* We are trending towards an early, pain filled death and a life full of sickness and disease if we do not permanently alter the way we think, eat, drink and carry out our lives.

Change yourself today, your community tomorrow and your world next week. Begin now, do *Revolutionary* acts by altering the way you see yourself and what you put into your body, soul and spirit. You can change the world once you change yourself.

TYPE II DIABETES

Risk factors or causes for becoming diabetic include, but are not limited to: being overweight or obese, sedentary lifestyle, unhealthy eating habits, high blood pressure and high cholesterol, alcohol consumption and depression.

Symptoms comprise increased thirst and frequent urination, increased hunger, weight loss, fatigue, blurred vision, slow healing of sores, frequent infections and areas of darkened skin.

In chapter 6, subsection Home Medical Equipment, point number five I mention you need a home blood glucose meter. I cannot stress this point enough! You must get a meter with the test strips and lancets and test your blood on a regular basis. Do this upon waking, before you eat or drink anything. Janie and I test our blood glucose levels on a regular basis.

To start, test your blood glucose levels every other day for two weeks and track your numbers. Armed with this data you have an average of your fasting blood glucose levels and now you can strategize how to keep your blood sugar levels balanced.

<u>WHAT TO DO ABOUT DIABETES</u>

To have *Revolutionary health* one must have a *Revolutionary* plan of action.

Paradigm Shifting was a title of a subsection of an earlier chapter. This is how you must view life to prevent diabetes (cancer, heart disease and other illnesses) or to put these illnesses into remission.

We must move beyond traditional ***and*** alternative medicines to, seemingly, radical *Revolutionary* techniques.

To prevent diabetes or to put it into remission you **must** change your lifestyle. In my book, *The 10-Day Total Body Revolution* I describe key factors that must be followed to achieve a total body transformation.

I recommend the reader purchase materials from the Selected Bibliography and References in the back of this book for materials that I have studied and glean wisdom in how to approach a new *Revolutionary* life.

PREVENTION AND REMISSION

To prevent or put into remission diabetes (cancer and heart disease) put into practice immediately the following practices:

1. Begin a modified Ketogenic lifestyle. You want the correct type and quantity of fats and proteins balanced with lots of vegetables and extremely low starchy carbohydrates (pasta, rice, potatoes, and bread). Research this type of life you that need to start living.
2. Lose weight. Print copies of the BMI chart which you can download and post it in your kitchen, workplace or wherever. If you are not in the healthy zone-the *Revolutionary* Zone-GET THERE. Being overweight or obese is the result of unhealthy eating and is the sign that a person will have severe health problems.

3. Get your soul healed of past wounds. Forgive who hurt you, let go of the pain, stop running, forgive yourself, do not hold a grudge, and make amends wherever you can. Live your life and be free from whatever past you had and look forward to a great future.

4. Get spicy and go herbal. In an upcoming section I will briefly describe a few spices and herbs you need to take daily.

5. Water. Drink your water. Stop all the sweet drinks. Consume MUCH less caffeine.

6. Exercise. Get my book *The 10-Day Total Body Revolution*, and see the bonus section included in this book.

7. Eat your vegetables. Lots and lots of green leafy vegetables. Raw, steamed, sautéed or stir fried-however you like (except covered in cheese) eat all types of colorful vegetables.

8. Utilize the medical equipment you purchased (from the previous chapter), get and know your numbers then make the changes you need to make in your life.

9. Find your motivational factors. Why do you want to be free from diabetes? For whom or what do you want to live free from disease?

Start today to send diabetes into remission or to never contract it in the first place. It is not impossible to be diabetes free. How much do you want remission? What are you willing to do to not stay or become diabetic?

GET SPICY & GO HERBAL

Amazing results have occurred for people who have begun to go spicy and herbal in their quest for *Revolutionary Health*. This section will be a quick review of a few herbs and spices you need every day, which have been scientifically studied, researched and proven to aid in achieving overwhelming, superior health. Do your own further extensive research to verify the claims presented here and then do not delay to "get spicy."

Olive Leaf Extract (OLE) is taken from the leaves of olive trees. It has been scientifically proven to balance blood glucose. There are many other benefits to taking OLE, just one is that it targets belly fat. I take 2,000 mg daily.

Cinnamon is proven to improve blood glucose numbers, triglycerides, LDL cholesterol, and total cholesterol. I use about a tablespoon of cinnamon daily in my oatmeal and coffee.

Ginseng, any variety is good to use. It has been studied for years and is proven to improve blood sugar control and glycosylated hemoglobin, which is monitored for our blood glucose levels. Taking 1,000 mg daily is great.

 Magnesium is needed to put diabetes into remission. It regulates blood sugar levels, needed for bone health, proper blood pressure, nerve function, and muscle formation and improves your immune system.

Aloe Vera is important to "smear" all over your skin. Traditionally used for burns and wounds on the skin, it soaks into our skin and helps to reduce blood glucose and glycosylated hemoglobin levels. Janie and I have lots of Aloe Vera plants in and around our home. I pinch off a stem and rub it all over my face and hands all the time. It has helped reduce my age spots, acne scars and lines under my eyes.

There are many other herbs and spices that you should start using immediately. If you begin with these you have a great start to improve your health and fight off rising blood sugar levels.

CONCLUSION

Diabetes can be prevented and put into remission! The only way is to seriously alter your lifestyle and beliefs then you will reap the benefits.

Investigate a modified Ketogenic lifestyle. Be cautious about consuming too many fats, the wrong types and too much protein without exercise. Check out the books I reference in the Bibliography.

Exercise, lose weight, track your numbers, eat garlic and go spicy. Forgive and let go of past wounds then your food addictions will start to fade away. Start OLE, cinnamon and ginseng immediately.

Do not forget your vegetables. Learn to like them if that is what you have to do. Learn how to prepare them in a variety of ways, watch Youtube videos of how people prepare their foods. Get your "colors on" by eating a wide variety of types and colors of vegetables.

Believe it or not, this is *Revolutionary* to most people. To take herbal supplements, forgive those who have hurt us, eat lots of vegetables, have the correct amount of fats and protein and of course eat an extremely less amount of empty carbohydrates and no more sugary sweet foods.

Step by step, day-by-day you will see the transformation in your life as you follow the procedures outlined in this chapter. You may notice quite soon, if you are diabetic, that you will need less of your medication due to your altered lifestyle as advocated here. I have seen this happen to many people, they have decreased to nearly eliminate all their diabetic medications as they increased their healthy, *Revolutionary*, habits.

This is how you put diabetes into remission. You can do it! Never Give Up, Never Give In, Never Say Die!

CHAPTER 11

CONCLUSION

Attaining *Revolutionary Health* is not easy, but it is not difficult. It is neither sorrowful nor relentless but is joyful and exciting. It is a time of self-reflection and a time of experimentation with novel concepts and techniques. It is *Revolutionary*.

I suggest you read this book again and then again. Take notes on the equipment to purchase and then go out and get what you need. Begin today to clean out your pantry and refrigerator of food and drink that is harmful. Begin today testing your taste buds with a wide variety of seed grains (quinoa, millet and others) and vegetables that you have not had previously (arugula, kale, butternut squash and others).

When you live the life of a *Revolutionary*, a radical "health nut", people will notice. Regardless of what your life was yesterday, today is a new day and you are not only turning a "new leaf" you are eating it!

Exercise with caution, yet get out there and start sweating and burn off those extra calories you have stored for perhaps years. Time for a change in your life and today is the day. The past is the past and you have a new, wonderful, healthy future waiting for you to put the key into the door and step on through to the other side of life.

You do not have to be overweight any longer, because you will never give in to negative thoughts or practices. You will achieve success because you will never give up. You are living a new life, full of energy, strength and vitality because you will never say die to your new rules for living and believing.

Go forward with your life, one BIG step immediately and smaller steps to follow every week. Believe in yourself. Know that you can accomplish anything you put your mind to doing and then get out there and do it. You are stronger than you realize.

Find a mentor or a support group to help, do not go it alone. If you have no one, contact me; let's see how we may be able to help. Life is too precious; YOUR life is too precious to not make it everything you are supposed to be!

There is much more detail to this *Revolutionary* lifestyle than can be covered in this short book. This is why I recommend my other book, *The 10-Day Total Body Revolution* and other books as noted in the Bibliography.

Reading and getting into these other books are great for reference, yet you must start on your own and decide **<u>YOU</u>** want to be disease free and put all these diseases into remission.

If you need help, contact me. I may be able to recommend a program in your area or give you encouragement when you cannot seem to take your life to the next level.

Start your *Revolutionary* journey today, one step at a time and one day at a time. In your new adventure, if and when you need a helping hand, reach out and grab hold of a mentor that can help.

So with that in mind, get motivated, start your metamorphosis, alter yourself and in so doing you will alter your environment.

Begin to change your life today. You are needed in this world and the world needs you!

Make a difference in society. Be the leader and great example you were born to be.

Never give up!
Never give in!
Never say die!

www.forerunnerspirit.com

SELECTED BIBLIOGRAPHY and REFERENCES

Holy Bible, New Living Translation, 2013, Carol Stream, Illinois, Tyndale House Publishers

Colbert, MD, Don, Dr. Colbert's Keto Zone Diet, 2017, Franklin, TN, Worthy Books

Colbert, MD, Don, Let Food Be Your Medicine: Dietary Changes Proven to Prevent and Reverse Disease, 2015, Franklin, TN, Worthy Books

Colbert, MD, Don. What You Don't Know May Be Killing You, 2004, Lake Mary, FL, Siloam, A Strang Company

Duke, James A, The Green Pharmacy, 1997, Emmaus, Pennsylvania, Rodale Press

Hyman, MD, Mark, Eat Fat, Get Thin: Why the Fat We Eat Is the Key to Sustained Weight Loss and Vibrant Health, 2016, Columbus GA, Little Brown & Company

Hyman, MD, Mark, The Blood Sugar Solution: The UltraHealthy Program for Losing Weight, Preventing Disease, and Feeling Great Now! 2014, Columbus GA, Little Brown & Company

Jakes, T. D., Lay Aside The Weight Taking Control of It Before It Takes Control of You! 1997, Tulsa, Albury Publishing.

Lerner, Ben, Body By God The Owner's Manual for Maximized Living, 2003, Nashville Tennessee, Thomas Nelson, Inc.

Loomis, James, The 10-Day Total Body Revolution, 2018, Atlanta Texas.

Loomis, James, Passionate Lover of God, 2018, Atlanta Texas.

Loomis, Janie, Spirit of the Forerunner: A Cry Goes Out, 2018, Atlanta Texas.

Monterey Bay Spice Company, www.herbco.com

1-800-500-6148, herbs, spices, teas and much more.

Chapter 3 of

James Loomis'

THE 10-DAY TOTAL BODY REVOLUTION

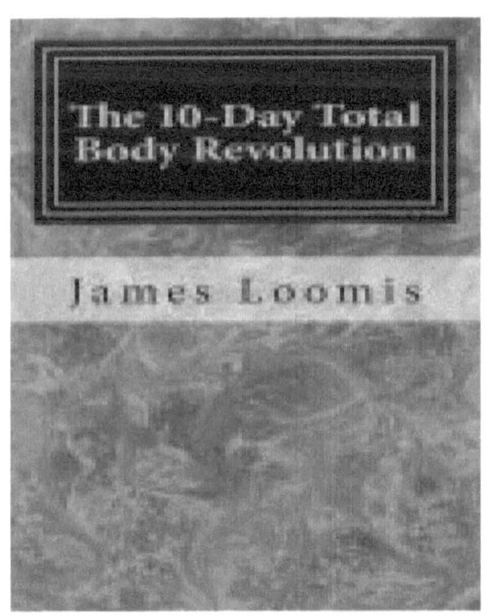

CHAPTER 3

EXERCISE: STRETCHING, AEROBIC, ANEROBIC & HIIT

Join a fitness center. Some centers are as inexpensive as $10.00 per month. Come on! You can afford $10.00; no more excuses! If you want to be a *Revolutionary*, you must revolutionize your body and the best way is through a fitness center. If you want a fitness trainer, utilize their expertise for your 10 days and extend the time if you so desire. Tell them what you are doing, how you want to improve and allow them to train you according to what you want. Push yourself. That is what this program is all about. Do what you have not done before to get results you have not had before.

<u>**STRETCHING**</u>

Begin each day by getting up earlier than you need for your daily activities and stretch. Go outside to the back porch, watch the sun rise, make room in your living room or wherever you have space and begin a routine of stretching exercises.

Have you observed cats or dogs and how they act after a time of sleep? They get up and stretch. It is natural for them to do so. Follow their example.

Stretch all your muscle groups. Internet search for pictures of stretching exercises if you like. Stand erect loosening your limbs, gently shaking out your arms and then each leg. Turn your head to the right then left, forward and backwards holding for 2-3 seconds each. Repeat procedure while raising and lowering your shoulders.

Extend your arms out sideways, palms down and reach as far as you can, hold for 5 seconds. Keep arms out and turn palms upward, hold for 5 seconds. Slowly raise your arms, keeping elbows straight and reaching fully until arms are straight above your head, palms touching, and hold 5 seconds. Reach right arm out forwards and left backwards. Hold and twist so palms face opposite directions, all the while reaching as far as you can. Extend and retract fingers as you hold your arms out.

Remain in the same standing position, stretch out arms from sides for balance and begin to lift one leg at a time forwards then backwards, hold for 5 seconds. Stretch your legs as far as you can. Stand with your back straight against the wall and raise one leg at a time up until parallel with the ground.

Now let's do some back stretching exercises. Lay on your back on the floor. Slowly raise one knee to your chest and hold for 5 to 10 seconds. Repeat using other leg. As you lay flat, twist your right leg over your left to be as perpendicular to your body as possible, hold then switch legs. Roll over onto your stomach, head up, elbows resting on floor sideways, pull your upper torso up so your palms are resting on the floor and you are arching your back, hold for 10 seconds. Get up to a sitting position, spread your legs, stretch your arms to hold your knees and slowly bend your head downward. Do not bend far, just enough so you can begin to feel a burn in your back.

Still in a sitting position, pull your legs back under your torso, stretch your arms forward over your head and bow your head to the floor. Hold for 5 to 10 seconds. Stay seated and raise your body back to a sitting position with arms raised up into the air over your head for 5 to 10 seconds. Repeat procedures three times.

There are numerous types of stretching exercises you can do. Start with these, if you have other favorites do those as well. The main objective is to spend at least 15 minutes daily stretching, if you are able to spend more time that is great; remember you are a *revolutionary* and everything is changing in your life!

AEROBIC EXERCISES

Types of aerobic exercises include, but not limited to spin bike, walking, swimming, jogging, treadmill walking, elliptical equipment, dancing, bicycle riding, cross county skiing, kickboxing and many others.

The type of "cardio" workout you are striving for is to get your heart beating faster. As you push yourself you feel yourself getting out of breath, your heart begins to pound and you sweat!

Start out with at least 20 minutes then work your way up to at least 30 minutes daily. This is all about shocking your body into a radical transformation and to do so you must push yourself. As noted on the copyright page, if you are under the care of a physician for a particular illness or condition, consult with your doctor as you begin a new program.

If you have NEVER done anything like this previously, now is the time to start your Revolution! You will start losing weight as you exercise, but will lose even more as your completely modify your eating and drinking habits.

<u>ANEROBIC EXERCISES</u>

Weight training is essential to your reformation. Talk to your trainer or someone at the gym about what you want and need toned. You need strong knees so work your leg muscles to strengthen your stance. You lose weight through overall working out (and especially through your changed eating and drinking habits), but increase your core strengthening to lose the fat around your belly, hips and thighs.

Work your arms and shoulders. We all need upper body strength. You need the strength and stamina to carry loads and go about your daily activities, regardless what you do you must strengthen your body. Ask questions at the center about the different weight training machines and free weights.

For the first 2 days, push, but get comfortable with the workout; then kick it up for the next 8 days. You should be on the weights for at least 30 minutes daily; increase to 45-60 minutes as you can. Yes, this is your new life; you work out and MAKE the time in your schedule to be healthy. This is the NEW you.

Do not give up. You are in a *Revolution*. This is your *Total Body Revolution*. This *Revolution* is accomplished through this aspect of exercise. Yes, every chapter in this book is key to your success, yet you have got to exercise if you want to see results.

HIIT

High-Intensity Interval Training is a type of workout that alternates between intense bursts of activity and fixed periods of less intense activity. These types of workouts can be done in or out of the fitness center.

Examples of HIIT are biking as fast as you can for 2 minutes then going slow for 5 minutes. Running as fast as you can for 30 seconds then walking for 5 minutes. Push yourself hard on the elliptical machine for 2 minutes then go slow for 10 minutes.

There are endless variations of this type of training and the benefits are astronomical! You can utilize this style of workout with any exercise routine. Use this method every other day allowing your body to recover in-between if you are really pushing yourself.

HIIT is great for cardio vascular training, fat burning and strengthening your heart. You can use equipment but it is not necessary. As you increase your metabolism to do these routines more often and longer, you can do this training anywhere and anytime and it is extremely challenging if you push yourself.

There are any number of exercises you can do: running, sprints, jumping, swimming, running in place, lifting, crunches, oblique crunches, stationary bike, regular bike riding, push ups, jumping jacks, burpee, jump rope, planking, high knee lifts, squat jumps, lunges, stair stepper, battle rope and so much more.

<u>CONCLUSION</u>

Gear up to work out! Your *Revolution* consists of exercise, altered food and drink choices, soul healing and thinking modification. Every aspect is co-dependant upon the other and a *Total Body Revolution* cannot be attained without each factor transfigured. Work out, work out hard, sweat and begin to feel your muscles ache. As you incorporate every aspect of your *Revolution*, you begin to feel changes throughout your body, soul and mind. You can do it! You must do it to be the *Revolutionary* that **everyone** around you needs you to be. Be an example setter of your revolutionary new lifestyle. Be the leader that you are and were created to be. Get ready for your new you!

ABOUT THE AUTHOR

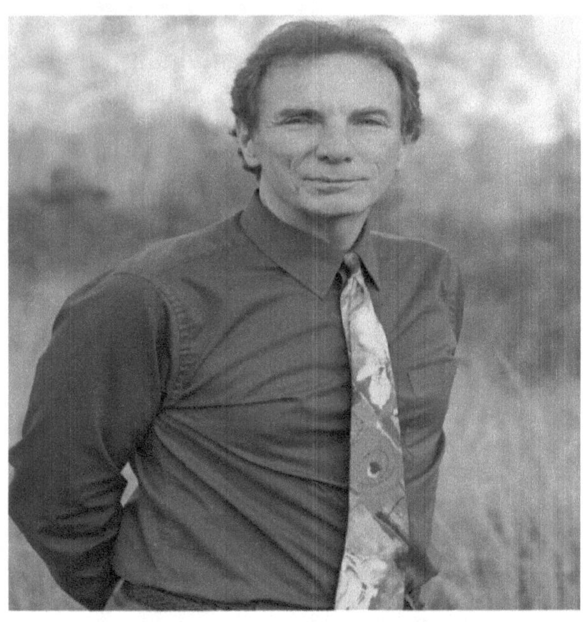

James Loomis is an auditor, a health and wellness columnist, nutritional researcher and a passionate lover of God. His health and wellness lectures are bold, hard hitting, fact and science based and convicting to all who want to hear the truth and learn how to become healthy and drug free. He and his wife Janie have been organic micro-farmers, gourmet foods manufacturers and marketers.

James and Janie are public speakers in secular and Christian seminars, are life-coaches, authors and fitness and health food fanatics.

James speaks with fire and conviction, humor and sensitivity on how to change one's circumstances and achieve personal success in every arena of life. He has seen countless people change their health through his instructions and lifestyle leadership in nutritional education.

He and Janie live in Atlanta, Texas.

Author photography by Elizabeth Howe of Fresh Wind Photography

Books by James and Janie Loomis are available via attending one of their conferences or seminars, through Amazon and on the website:

www.forerunnerspirit.com

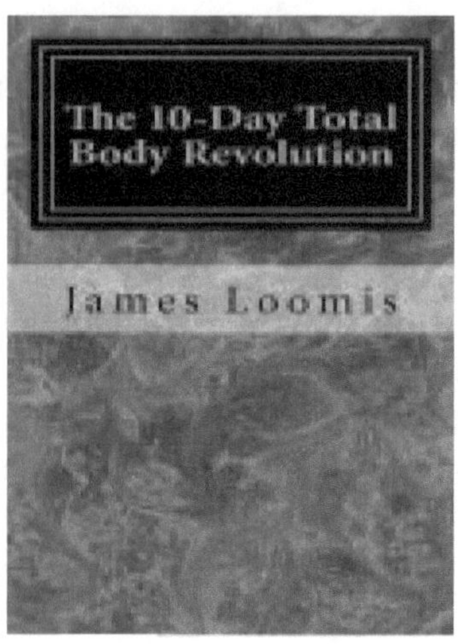

The 10-Day Total Body Revolution is:

* ❖ A guide to encourage your renovation into superior health.
* ❖ The step-by-step process to undertake for the beginning of the rest of your life.
* ❖ Reveals truths that free your heart from past wounds.
* ❖ Educates on the value of food choices and preparation techniques.
* ❖ Gives you confidence to pursue your life goals.
* ❖ Provides easy to follow lifestyle examples.
* ❖ Illustrates practical guidelines how to purge toxins from your body.
* ❖ Goes beyond tradition to illustrate breakthrough techniques you can apply from day one for complete life changing, soul healing and mind transformation.

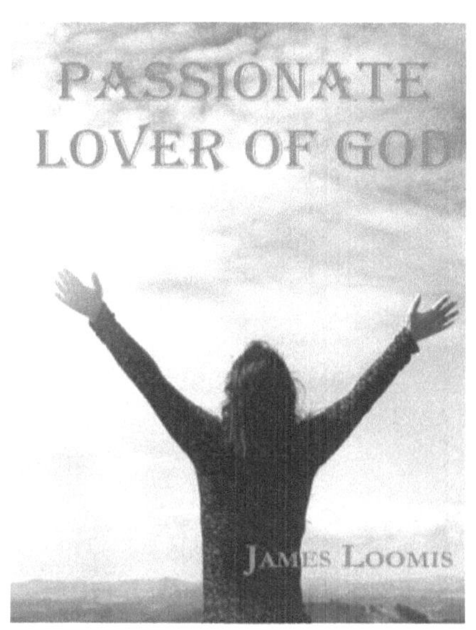

PASSIONATE LOVER OF GOD is:

--The tool you need to grow closer to God
--Your EVANGELISTIC tool to reach your world
    for Jesus
--The clarion call that awakens us to a deeper
    relationship with God
--The step-by-step guide you will want to share
    with everyone
--The clear point-by-point explanation on how to
    walk out your new intimate relationship
    with God
--Full of relatable life stories and easy reading
--YOUR mandate to draw intensely, passionately
    in love with Jesus
--The Bride of Christ cleansing herself for her
    soon wedding

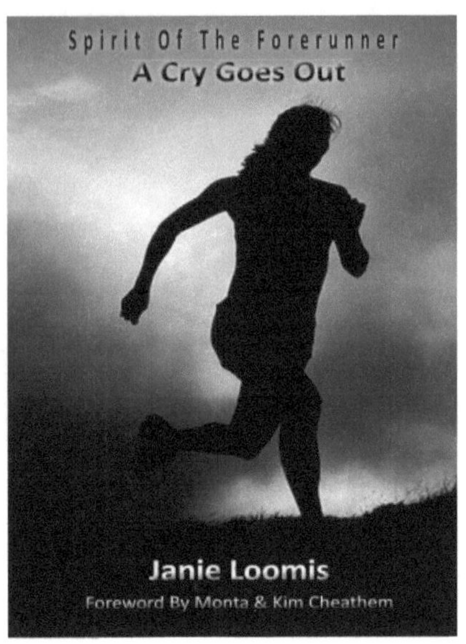

Spirit of the Forerunner: A Cry Goes Out

Intercession is a vital key to the prayer life of the Forerunner.
As Forerunners, we are to help the body of Christ understand their place on the world scene.
Forerunners are deeply prophetic and take very seriously the prophetic call on their lives.

As we draw closer to God in our worship, we begin to see as He sees, touch as He touches and know what He knows.

When we draw close to Him, we hear His heart.

The Legacy Of One Who Has Gone Before

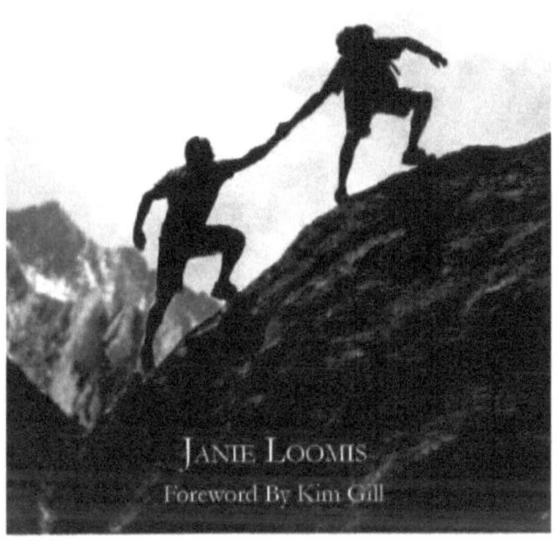

Spirit of the Forerunner: The Legacy Of One Who Has Gone Before

It is only through an obedient and humble spirit that
God can use us for His glory.
If you are holding on to a word or promise from God,
become obstinate, resolute and firm in belief that the
promise is coming about and it is
God's will to be done!
The key is our stepping out in faith. Have you taken a
"leap of Faith"?
The Forerunner has been called and
anointed by God to speak
for the Father, use your voice, speak with the
authority He has placed upon your calling.
People will see the anointing on your life
and be drawn to it.

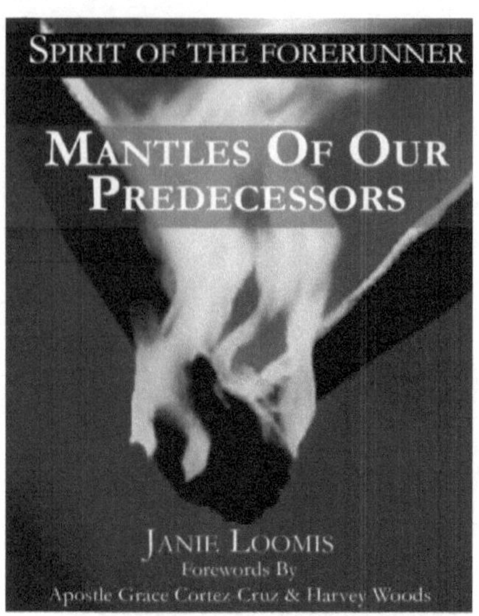

Spirit of the Forerunner:
Mantles of Our Predecessors

When you walk in the anointing of the forerunner, Holy Spirit causes the fire of God to consume people. Think beyond impossible and shake heaven and earth for the sake of your call.

Lock your eyes on the prize and look with spiritual understanding into your future.

This, the final book within the spirit of the Forerunner series, completes the calling and enables you to step out under the power and anointing given to the forerunner. As you walk cloaked with the mantle of our predecessors, you will gain confidence in your vocation and understand the importance of the forerunner in God's kindgom plan.

9 781731 556448